Concise Guide to
Respiratory Disease in the Horse

———— Concise Guide to ————
Respiratory Disease in the Horse

David W. Ramey, DVM

Trafalgar Square Publishing
North Pomfret, Vermont

First published in 2004 by
Trafalgar Square Publishing
North Pomfret, Vermont 05053

Printed in the United States of America

Disclaimer
This book is not to be used in place of veterinary care and expertise. The author and publisher shall have neither liability nor responsibility to any person or entity with respect to any loss or damage caused or alleged to be caused directly or indirectly by the information contained in this book. While the book is as accurate as the author can make it, there may be errors, omissions, and inaccuracies.

Library of Congress Cataloging-in-Publication Data

Ramey, David W.
  A concise guide to respiratory disease in the horse / David W. Ramey.
     p. cm.
  ISBN 1-57076-294-5 (pbk.)
  1. Horses--Diseases. 2. Respiratory organs--Diseases. I. Title.
  SF959.R47R27 2004
  636.1'08962--dc22

                                        2004013153

Illustrations by Robert Amaral
Typeface: Leawood and Sabon

10 9 8 7 6 5 4 3 2 1

CONTENTS

Acknowledgments　　vii

Introduction　　ix

CHAPTER 1
Anatomy and Physiology　1

CHAPTER 2
Diagnostic Techniques for Respiratory Problems　13

CHAPTER 3
Medical Treatments　23

CHAPTER 4
Upper Airway Problems　35

CHAPTER 5
Lower Airway Problems　43

CHAPTER 6
Pleuropneumonia ("Shipping Fever")　51

CHAPTER 7
Streptococcus equi Infection ("Strangles")　59

CHAPTER 8
Inflammatory Disease of the Lower Airway ("Heaves")　69

CHAPTER 9
Exercise-Induced Pulmonary Hemorrhage ("Bleeding")　81

Afterword　87

Bibliography　88

Index　90

ACKNOWLEDGMENTS

I have always been very fortunate to have many people help me make sure that the information provided in my books is up-to-date and accurate. I am not so bold as to consider myself an "expert" in each and every area about which I write, however, I am lucky enough to know many people who are. Some of those people have been extremely generous and willing to lend their time and expertise to reviewing some, or all, of this book.

Mike Davis, DVM, PhD, Associate Professor of Equine Medicine at Oklahoma State University's School of Veterinary Medicine, looked over the chapters on heaves, shipping fever, and anatomy and physiology. In addition to helping people understand the horse's respiratory system, Dr. Davis is doing some fascinating work on sled dogs and their GI system. A renaissance man of medicine, as it were.

Tom Goetz, DVM, DACVIM, Professor of Equine Medicine & Surgery, Department of Veterinary Clinical Medicine at the College of Veterinary Medicine of the University of Illinois, was kind enough to review the chapter on EIPH. His work has been invaluable in helping veterinarians understand this difficult condition.

Philip Johnson, MRCVS, PhD, Associate Professor of Equine Medicine at the University of Missouri's School of Veterinary Medicine, reviewed the chapter on diagnostic techniques for respiratory disease. It truly is amazing what can be done to try to figure out what's wrong with a horse's breathing apparatus when capable hands, such as Dr. Johnson's, are engaged.

Pam Wilkins, a Professor of Equine Medicine at the University of Pennsylvania School of Veterinary Medicine, was kind enough to review the chapter on lower airway diseases. She's authored articles in many texts on the subject and shepherded many students through the horse's respiratory system. I am lucky to have had her help and encouragement, not only in this, but other important areas. I can never thank her enough.

Nat Messer, DVM, DABVP, Associate Professor of Equine Medicine and Surgery at the University of Missouri graciously reviewed the chapter on medications. A former professor of mine, I am lucky enough to keep learning from him.

Eric Reinertson, DVM, Professor of Equine Medicine and Surgery and head of the Department of Large Animal Medicine at Iowa State University, reviewed the chapter on upper airway problems. Pragmatic and practical, I was fortunate to train with him for a year after veterinary school. His influence endures.

John Madigan, MS, DVM, Professor of Equine Medicine and Epidemiology at the University of California, Davis, reviewed the chapter on strangles, a controversial topic if ever there was one. His erudition, tempered with a great sense of humor, are continuing gifts to veterinarians everywhere.

Valerie Devaney, DVM, and Mike Graper, DVM, are good friends that consented to read the whole book, so as to make sure that it seemed practical. Valerie's Mom made sure that it was comprehensible to the audience for which the book is intended. Hilary Brown, who doesn't own horses, said that she could understand it, too. Thanks to you all.

Finally, to Jackson and Aidan, and to watching you grow. I wish that time wasn't passing so quickly, but you sure do seem to be headed in the right direction.

INTRODUCTION

The respiratory tract of the horse is an intricate, important, and sometimes difficult body system to treat. After problems with the horse's gastrointestinal tract, medical problems affecting the various parts of the breathing apparatus undoubtedly make up the next most common of all medical conditions affecting the horse. From a simple cough to horses that bleed from their lungs when exercised, from newborn babies to geriatrics, the horse's respiratory tract often presents dilemmas for veterinarians and horse owners alike (not to mention the horses).

Over the years, much has been learned about the diagnosis and treatment of respiratory conditions of the horse. Of course, there's still a lot that has to be learned, but proper handling and management can prevent or lessen the signs of many conditions. With modern medical treatments, those that haven't been prevented can often be managed to a successful outcome.

Chapter 1 takes you on a trip through the horse's respiratory tract, showing you what the tract does and where problems might occur. Chapter 2 introduces you to the diagnostic methods that are used to differentiate the most common conditions that affect the horse's breathing system. Chapter 3 then moves on to discuss the most common treatments for those conditions. The subsequent chapters examine some of the more common problems of the horse's respiratory system that are likely to be encountered. With knowledge comes understanding.

Anatomy and Physiology

Rational diagnostic and treatment schemes are derived from approaches that are based on working with the horse's body. It's not really accurate to say that medicine "cures" medical conditions, rather, rational treatments, properly applied, set up situations that allow the horse's body to return to normal (or as close to normal as possible). So, in order to properly apply medical therapies to the horse's respiratory system, it's important to know a good bit about the structures that make up the system and what they do. Knowing that, you can target therapies to help the horse's breathing apparatus do its job.

Imagine that you're an air molecule, heading into a horse. You've got quite a journey ahead of you. You're going to be passing through and by a number of very important structures. Ultimately, your fate is to be used by the horse to assist in his normal body functions. Here's a travelogue of the sights you'll see along the way (the anatomy) and the reasons that you're taking this trip in the first place (the physiology).

NOSTRILS

Your journey inside the horse starts as you pass through one of the horse's *nostrils*. The horse has to breathe through his nose—he can't breathe through his mouth like you can because of the configuration of his larynx, deep in his throat. The nostrils are the external openings to the horse's respiratory tract. The horse can open his nostrils wider when he needs to take in more air, such as when he exercises.

From a disease diagnosis standpoint, you'll mostly notice what's coming *out* of your horse's nostrils. The passage is open to travel in both directions.

NASAL PASSAGES

After you breeze by the nostrils, you will go up a rigid tube. There are two of these, one set on each side of the horse's head. The horse's *nasal passages* are divided into three channels, and each is lined with a mucous membrane that's full of blood vessels (fig. 1). As the nasal passages come to an end, just before they open into the horse's pharynx, you'll encounter the *ethmoturbinate bones*—small, spongy bones that are tightly rolled up, like a scroll. If you could lay the surfaces of these bones out flat, you'd find that they cover a remarkably large surface area.

The mucous membranes of the nasal passage perform several important functions for the horse. These include warming, filtering, and humidifying the air that the horse breathes. And, the nasal passage is the first line of defense against invading organisms, bringing the breathed-in air in contact with mucus-coated membranes that contain immune factors. Air that the horse breathes in contacts the nerves of smell that line the nasal passage, as well.

SINUSES

Inside the horse's head are several *sinuses* that are directly connected into the nasal passages by small passageways. A sinus is just a big space, lined with a mucous membrane that most likely helps to warm and moisten the air that the horse breathes.

Sinuses are not often a problem for the horse. However, sometimes, respiratory infection can block normal sinus drainage, and the sinuses can become infected, resulting in a condition called *sinusitis*. In addition, the upper-teeth roots open into the sinuses, and infection of a tooth root can extend into a sinus.

The exact function of the sinus is not clear in the horse (or, in any species). There are a number of theories as to its function, including adding resonance to vocalization, equalizing pressure differences within the nasal cavity, helping to condition inhaled air, protecting structures inside the head from trauma, and reducing the weight of the skull without sacrificing its strength.

PALATE

The *palate*, known to the ancient Greeks as the "diaphragm of the mouth" (*diaphragma oris*), separates the oral passage from the nasal

FIGURE 1

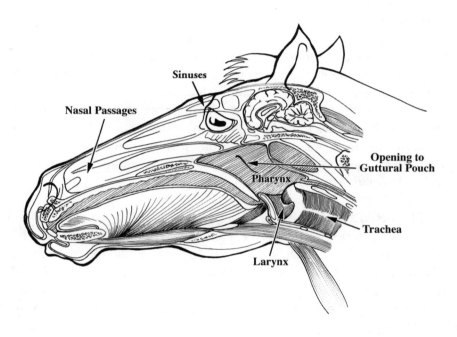

The major structures of the respiratory tract include the nasal passages, guttural pouches, sinuses, pharynx, larynx, and trachea.

passages. Since you're an air molecule, you get to pass above the bony hard palate, which forms the floor of the nasal passages (above) and the roof of the mouth (below). The palate that extends beyond the bone forms the soft portion of the palate. For the horse, the back of the soft palate forms an intricate mechanism that's critical for normal breathing and swallowing (which is further discussed later in this chapter).

PHARYNX

Leaving the nasal passage, you now enter a chamber called the *pharynx*, or more commonly, the throat (see fig. 1). In the pharynx, air coming through the nostrils enters the same area as food does when it comes through the mouth (curiously, the ancient Greeks believed that secretions from the brain poured directly into the pharynx, but modern medicine has moved beyond such ideas). The pharynx of the horse can become inflamed due to dust or allergy, resulting in a condition called *pharyngitis*. More importantly, some critical structures open into this chamber.

GUTTURAL POUCHES

Just after entering the pharynx, you (the air molecule) will pass by two "slits," one on each side of you. If you imagine the pharynx as the face of a clock, the slits are positioned at about ten o'clock and two o'clock—a little over half-way up each side of the chamber. These slits are the openings to the horse's *guttural pouches* (see fig. 1). The equine guttural pouch is a large, air-filled sac of the ear tube, and the slits are actually openings where the horse's ear tubes meet his pharynx. People have the same sort of thing, and it allows them to equalize pressure on their ears, say, when diving under water or going up in the air in a plane.

In the horse, it appears that the guttural pouch may be important for brain cooling. Recent investigations suggest that, contrary to what was once believed, air does not pass in and out of the guttural pouch with each breath. Rather, researchers now believe that air can be taken into the guttural pouch when needed to ventilate and cool the large *internal carotid arteries* that pass through each pouch and directly to the horse's brain. Experiments have shown that whenever the guttural pouches are ventilated with cooled or warmed environmental air, temperatures in the arteries drop. This sort of cooling mechanism would be especially important during heavy exercise when the horse needs to do everything he can to keep his body temperature down.

The guttural pouch can occasionally become a problem for the horse, most particularly when it is affected by one of various infectious agents. Sorting out problems with the guttural pouch can be a diagnostic and therapeutic challenge for your veterinarian (there's more information on them in chapter 4).

LARYNX

When you reach the lower rear portion of the pharynx, you will see a firm structure made up of cartilage and muscle and lined with the moist mucous membrane that is continuous throughout the horse's respiratory tract. The *larynx* connects the back part of the pharynx to the front part of the *trachea*, or windpipe (see fig. 1). It guards the entrance to the trachea and also functions as the organ of the horse's voice (without a larynx, there wouldn't be whinnying).

Two large, muscular cartilages, the *arytenoid cartilages*, front the horse's larynx. These cartilages close when the horse swallows, which allows food to go over the windpipe (rather than in) and down the esophagus. Conversely, when the horse needs extra air, the muscles of the cartilages contract, opening up the entrance to the trachea to its maximum diameter, acting much like the doors of an opening elevator.

The location of the nerve supply to the cartilage of the larynx, particularly along the left side, results in a condition that is relatively unique to the horse. On the left side, the nerve to the larynx—the *recurrent laryngeal nerve*—actually runs very close to the skin surface, just under the horse's jugular vein. In this location, it can be relatively easily damaged due to trauma or, unfortunately, inflammation caused by the injection of irritating substances that are intended to go in the jugular vein, but miss. When the nerve is damaged, the horse's larynx doesn't function properly and surgical solutions may be necessary. The horse's larynx can also become inflamed, resulting in *laryngitis*, and in rare instances, parts of the larynx, particularly the laryngeal cartilages, can become infected.

At the base of the horse's larynx is his *epiglottis*. The epiglottis is a tongue of cartilage that acts like a lid for the larynx. When the horse swallows, the epiglottis helps prevent food from going down the wrong pipe.

The important structures of the larynx, that is, the cartilages and the epiglottis, fit into the soft palate like a button in a buttonhole. This allows for an airtight seal when the horse breathes. This arrangement is unique to the horse, and it explains why a horse has to breathe through his nose. When a horse is really breathing hard, such as during exercise, he can't get any extra air by taking deep breaths through his mouth, like a person can, because the larynx is "buttoned" into the soft palate (fig. 2). Even when a horse appears to pant, such as after heavy exercise, it's all just tongue-flapping, to no avail!

Problems can occur for the horse when the soft palate becomes displaced to a position above the epiglottis. This is a condition called *dorsal displacement of the soft palate*. Normally, the "button" of the larynx fits in the "buttonhole" of the palate, except when the horse swallows, coughs, or whinnies. Because it causes a narrowing of the upper airways and/or soft palate flapping, a displaced palate is abnormal and makes it hard for the horse to breathe. This can be a problem during strenuous exercise and occurs most often in race-horses.

TRACHEA

Once you (the air molecule) have managed to pass by the epiglottis, you can celebrate because you've made it to the horse's *trachea*, or windpipe (see fig. 1). This is the tube that connects the *upper* air passages in the horse's head with the *lower* air passages in the horse's lungs. It's made up of a series of firm cartilage rings and looks very much like the hose that connects a home clothes dryer to an outside vent. Like the entire airway, the trachea is lined with a moist mucous membrane. It's also lined with little hairs, called *cilia*, which help move bacteria, mucus, and debris away from the lungs to where it can be breathed out, or swallowed.

While not often a problem in and of itself, the trachea can occasionally become inflamed, particularly in a horse with *allergic airway disease*. This results in a condition called *tracheitis*.

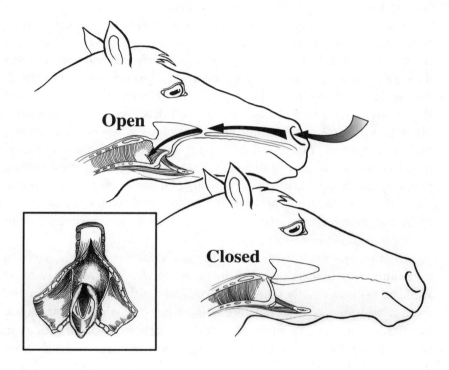

FIGURE 2

Open

Closed

*The horse only breathes through the nose because of the airtight seal
that is created by the "button" of the larynx fitting into the
"buttonhole" of the soft palate.*

LUNGS

The two *lungs* of the horse are the organs of respiration. Unlike other mammals, horse lungs aren't separated into lobes; rather, each lung is one large structure. A thin, watery coating, known as the *pleura*, covers the outer surface of each lung. Within the lung itself, air molecules, like you, move deeper and deeper until they reach the terminal respiratory units, the *alveoli*, where the most important function of the lung, gas exchange, occurs.

The critical function of the horse's lung is to exchange oxygen from the air for carbon dioxide (a by-product of the body's metabolism) from the blood. The balance between oxygen and carbon dioxide is rather precisely controlled and rather obviously managed. Problems affecting the lung can affect the delivery of oxygen to, and the removal of carbon dioxide from, the horse's body. So, for example, when a horse needs more oxygen, such as when he's exercising, the horse breathes faster and more deeply so as to take in more oxygen. In certain disease conditions, or when a lung is not functioning properly, carbon dioxide can build up. Under such circumstances, the horse's respiration rate will go up, as well. Indeed, one of the most common signs of disease of the horse's respiratory tract is an increase in the respiration rate.

Defense against invading disease agents such as bacteria, viruses, and fungi is provided by the horse's *mucociliary system*. Mucus— well, snot—is normally secreted by the cells of the lung. It's removed from the lung by the hairlike *cilia* that line the air passages. Normally, this arrangement prevents the accumulation of mucus in the air passages. When the air passages are irritated, from disease, infection, or surface irritants, for example, mucus secretion increases. The mucus is removed from the air passages and eventually shows up in the horse's nostrils, hence, the snotty nose. Accumulations of mucus in the air passages interfere with lung function and, unfortunately, can be a problem in some disease processes.

Of course, the horse's lungs have other important functions. The lungs also serve to help the horse lose body heat through a process called *evaporative cooling*. Evaporative cooling is the same physics that cools your cup of hot tea. In hot tea, the most energetic water molecules escape from the cup as steam. When they do this, they take away more than their share of heat, and the atoms left behind in the cup are colder because they have lost energy. So it is in the horse, where the hottest molecules leave his body first, cooling him off in the process. As a result, in hot climates, or after heavy exercise, the horse breathes a bit faster than normal.

BRONCHI

The *bronchi* (one bronchus, two or more bronchi) are the air passages that will take you deep into the horse's lungs. Rigid structures, and much like tree branches in their configuration, bronchi go deeper and deeper into the lung, allowing air molecules to penetrate down to the level of the alveolus, most fundamental unit of the lung. Bronchi become inflamed in many respiratory diseases of the horse. Inflammation of the bronchi is called *bronchitis*.

ALVEOLI

Finally, your journey reaches the smallest chamber in the lung, the *alveolus* (fig. 3). An alveolus is a small, many-sided, sac-like structure. It's here that gas exchange takes place. When brought together in the optimum amounts, oxygen and carbon dioxide move between the air and the blood by a process known as *diffusion*—the oxygen and carbon dioxide molecules move back-and-forth spontaneously, and extra work is not required from the horse's body.

BLOOD VESSELS

There are actually two blood circulations to the horse's lungs. Most of the blood flow is involved with the important functions of gas exchange. There's also another circulation—*bronchial circulation*—that provides nutrients to the airways, lungs, and pleura, about which very little is known. However, the *pulmonary circulation*—the collection of blood vessels from which gas is exchanged—becomes involved in a condition known as *exercise-induced pulmonary hemorrhage*, which is the subject of chapter 9.

MUSCLES OF RESPIRATION

The *muscles of respiration* work to increase and decrease the volume of the horse's chest cavity. Breathing in—increasing the volume of the chest cavity—is called *inspiration*, and breathing out—decreasing the volume—is called *expiration*. In horses, like most mammals,

FIGURE 3

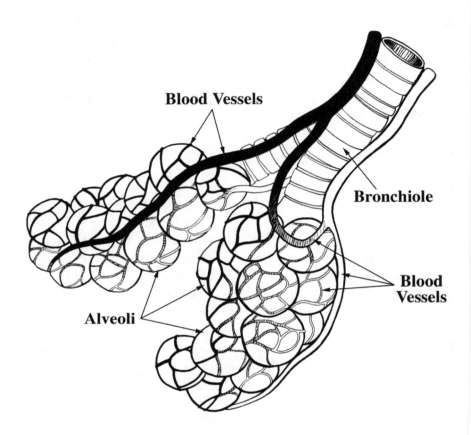

Blood Vessels

Bronchiole

Blood Vessels

Alveoli

The oxygen and carbon dioxide exchange takes place in the alveolus, the smallest chamber in the lung.

the most important muscles of inspiration are the *diaphragm* (a thin, flat muscle that separates the chest from the abdomen) and the *intercostal muscles* (the muscles that lie between the horse's ribs). These muscles work together to expand the horse's chest cavity, allowing air to flow into the lungs.

The horse's *abdominal muscles* are mainly responsible for expiration (that is, they help the horse push air out of his lungs). When the abdominal muscles contract, they force the diaphragm forward and decrease the volume of the horse's chest, pushing the air out in the process.

PLEURA

There is a thin, continuous membrane that lines the lung, as well as the chest cavity, on each side of the horse's body. This membrane is called the *pleura*. The pleura is moistened by a watery secretion that helps the lungs slide against the chest wall during breathing. The lung and chest-wall pleura thus form a potential space called the *pleural cavity*. It's a "potential space" because in the normal horse, the two sides touch each other and there isn't any space between them. Still, they are two separate surfaces.

The watery, pleural fluid between the chest wall and each lung keeps the lung from being pulled away from the chest wall and allows for normal breathing. Here's how it works. Imagine that you put a glass microscope slide, with a handle, on top of another glass slide. If you pull up on the handle, the top slide lifts up. But if you put a little bit of water between the two slides, lifting the upper one will lift the lower one, too. This is because there's now negative pressure between the two glass slides. Now imagine that the lower slide is attached to a rubber band, which is attached to a desk. That gives the system elasticity. That is, the system is flexible and can return to its initial state after you stretch it.

The relationship between the chest wall and the lung is similar to this example. The lung is like the lower slide with the rubber band attached to it. The chest wall is like the upper slide with the handle. There is water between the chest wall and lung, produced by the pleura. The water keeps the two surfaces together. The inward elastic force of the lung works to push air out. The outward elastic force of the chest wall, assisted by the pull of the muscles of breathing, works to expand the chest wall and lung and take air in.

The pleural surfaces can become involved in disease processes in the horse, especially when a horse is transported and develops a condition known as "shipping fever." It's a topic that's so important, it deserves its own chapter!

Understanding the structure and function of the horse's lungs is crucial to understanding respiratory disease, how to diagnose it, and how to treat it. The next chapter describes many of the important tools used in diagnosis.

2

Diagnostic Techniques for Respiratory Problems

Disease of the horse's respiratory tract is one of the most frequently seen medical problems by those who work with horses. Fortunately, many routine cases get better without a whole lot of fuss. In addition, the horse's respiratory tract is relatively user-friendly in terms of the diagnostic process. That is, if some part of the tract is diseased, or isn't working properly, it is fairly accessible and there are a lot of different tools that a veterinarian can use to evaluate it.

However, the horse's respiratory tract is rather limited in the ways it can actually indicate that something is wrong. In other words, there are only a few common clinical signs that can tell you there is a problem with the tract, but there are many, very different possible problems. So, for example, you may become aware of the fact that there's a problem with your horse's respiratory tract because he has a cough, but from that point, your veterinarian may need to turn to more complicated procedures in an effort to find out exactly what the problem is.

HISTORY
Even though there are all sorts of fancy procedures that can be used to evaluate the horse's breathing apparatus, there's just no substitute for talking with your veterinarian about what's been going on with your horse. So, part of diagnosing your horse's respiratory problem is going to involve discussing such things as how long it's been going on, how many horses in the farm or stable may have the same problem, how the horses have responded to previous treatments, recent activities (say, travel), or other problems that may be going on at the same time. Maybe you heard coughing, or you noticed an unusual

breathing noise coming from your horse when he's running. Maybe he's had a runny nose, from one or both nostrils. Perhaps he hasn't been exercising normally or he tires easily. Other questions can give vital clues to what's going on. For example, have any vaccines been given? Have any new horses entered your horse's environment? What's that environment like, anyway? Is it dusty, or is the hay of poor quality? Often, such information can give your veterinarian a good idea about what's going on before he or she even starts to examine the horse.

PHYSICAL EXAMINATION

Once all of the talking is over and you've given your veterinarian your best information about what's been going on, it's time to let your veterinarian get to work. He is going to compare your horse to all of the normal horses that he has seen or learned about.

You can learn a lot about your horse just by looking at him. The normal resting breathing rate for an adult horse ranges from 12 to 24 breaths per minute, and it may be up to 40 breaths per minute in a young foal. Often, when a horse has a respiratory problem, he'll breathe faster than normal, trying, for example, to get in air or blow off the accumulated body heat from a fever. He may be breathing with difficulty and with nostrils flaring—these are all important things to assess.

The presence of nasal discharge can be a good clue as to what's going on with your horse's respiratory tract. Normally, the tract secretes mucus that is swallowed and rarely seen. However, in disease, the respiratory tract—which is rather limited in the things that it can do to respond to problems—produces excessive secretions. Gravity can be your friend here—many times, nasal discharge is more evident when the horse's head is lowered, such as when he eats off the ground. The characteristics of the stuff coming out of your horse's nose can be useful in determining a diagnosis. What color is it—white, or red, or green, or yellow, or black? Is it coming from one or both sides? What is its nature (is it thick or watery)? What does it smell like? (Not that any of it smells good, but certain problems, such as bad teeth or diseased lung tissue, can also cause a nasal discharge that can really smell bad.)

You'll also want to look for any other external signs of a problem. One that everyone seems to look for is swelling between the jaws, which can be a sign of *Streptococcus equi* infection ("strangles"). But, other external signs can indicate disease, as well, and might not be as obvious: for example, swelling in the facial area could indicate a sinus infection, or discolored gums might indicate that a horse is having trouble getting enough oxygen into his body.

A thermometer is a really handy tool when working on a horse with respiratory problems. A horse's normal resting temperature is between 99.5 and 101 degrees Fahrenheit (37.5 to 38.3 degrees Celsius). Usually—but not always—when a horse has signs of a respiratory problem and his temperature increases, it's a sign that there's some sort of an infection in his body. The amount of fever does not necessarily correlate with how sick the horse is, however. In fact, horses tend to have fevers that are fairly high, relative to normal, because their body size makes it hard for them to get rid of heat. For example, if your horse is sick and has a fever of 104 degrees Fahrenheit, don't panic, but do call your veterinarian.

The other indispensable tool for the diagnosis of respiratory disease is a *stethoscope*. A stethoscope is simply an instrument that helps you listen to the sounds inside the horse's body. It's a rather old tool (the stethoscope was invented by the French physician R.T.H. Laënnec—who is considered to be the "father of chest medicine"—in 1816) but an incredibly useful one. Using a stethoscope, your veterinarian can explore your horse's chest and find all sorts of interesting audible clues as to what's going on, from the wheezes and crackles that characterize some types of *allergic airway disease* to the gurgles and congestion that can accompany infection. Sometimes, *no* sounds are heard, which can indicate, for example, that there's fluid in the chest (muffling the sounds) or that a lung is full of fluid and not inflating normally (as may happen with *pneumonia*). Respiratory sounds have even been recorded and analyzed, and some conditions of the horse's upper air passages demonstrated unique sound patterns that may be useful in diagnosis. Of course, it takes a bit of training to do any of this, but that's what veterinary schools are for!

Often, your veterinarian may use some sort of a "rebreathing apparatus" when examining your horse's airways. Plastic bags, rectal palpation sleeves, or even plastic foot boots can be placed over the horse's muzzle to force the horse to rebreathe the air that he exhales. Making the horse rebreathe his exhaled carbon dioxide results in a faster and deeper respiratory pattern as the horse's carbon dioxide intake gets higher and higher and the oxygen content of his blood gets lower and lower. Putting a bag over the horse's muzzle is a great way to make abnormal noises in the horse's chest sound louder. And, since the horse won't breathe deeply on command (as you can do for your doctor), it's about the only practical way to get it done without making the horse exercise. An abnormal horse may cough when forced to take deep breaths, get restless or appear distressed very quickly, or take a long time to return to a normal breathing pattern once the bag is removed. This technique, however, poses no threat to the horse (although some horses may not like a plastic bag waving around their muzzle).

The presence of a cough can give a clue as to what might be going on. As mentioned, if a horse coughs when forced to take deep breaths, something's likely to be wrong. But not all coughs come from deep in the horse's chest. For example, dust and smoke can irritate a horse's air passages, and in such cases, the horse can sometimes be made to cough if you squeeze the sides of his windpipe together.

During an examination, your veterinarian is likely to be looking around at many other things, such as the stabling conditions and feed quality, which give clues as to why a problem might have occurred in the first place. In the same vein, he is going to be looking at other parts of the horse, in addition to the respiratory tract, because sometimes problems in one area can be accompanied by problems in another area. For example, *laminitis* can be a complication of severe chest infection and *heart disease* can cause coughing. *Anhidrosis*, a failure to sweat usually seen in hot, humid climates, can cause increased respiratory effort, exercise intolerance, overheating, and a watery nasal discharge—all signs that can be easily mistaken for respiratory infection. It's important not to forget that there's a whole horse attached to those lungs!

Blood Sampling

Routine blood tests are often useful in helping to determine the type and extent of a horse's respiratory problem. When a horse has an infection of his air passages, *white blood cells*, the cells that the horse's body recruits to help fight off infection, typically increase in number, (although blood counts may be normal even in the face of infection).

The degree to which the number of white blood cells increases or decreases can be a useful indicator of how bad things really are. In the case of acute and severe infection, white blood cells may initially decrease because the demand for them exceeds the supply: the white blood cells may go to the infection from the bloodstream faster than the body can replace them in the blood. Levels of *inflammatory proteins* may rise with airway disease—these can be measured, as well. If the disease has been going on for some time, low *red blood cell* counts that occur due to chronic disease may develop, called *anemia*. These anemias don't need any special treatment—they get better when the horse gets better. Blood tests can also evaluate the condition of other body systems that may be compromised by the horse's respiratory problem.

While perhaps not a common diagnostic tool, particularly in field practice, blood from surface arteries can also be sampled to see how much oxygen is in it. A horse with severe airway problems can't get normal amounts of oxygen into his blood. Measuring blood gases can also help evaluate the response to treatment—normal blood oxygen levels should return as the horse's condition improves.

Endoscopy

Fiberoptic technology allows veterinarians to look directly at the horse's respiratory tract. Veterinarians can put an *endoscope* just about anywhere in the respiratory tract (fig. 4). They can look easily at such structures as the nasal passages, the guttural pouches, the larynx, the epiglottis, and the trachea—even down into the lungs with a long enough scope. If necessary, the veterinarian can cut a small hole in a place such as one of the horse's sinuses or his chest cavity to put the scope in and have a look. Such direct examination is a great way to confirm a diagnosis that may be suspected after the history and physical examination.

In a hospital situation, a horse can be examined with an endoscope while he is actively exercising on a treadmill. This exam is

FIGURE 4

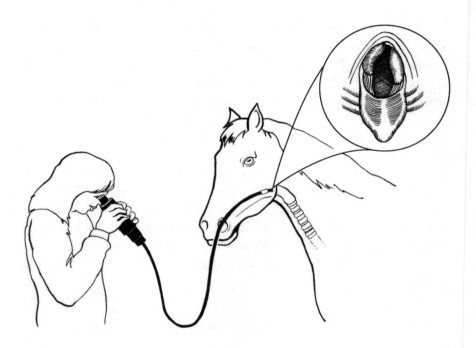

The endoscope allows the veterinarian to look directly at the horse's respiratory tract.

very useful when evaluating a horse with performance problems or that makes funny noises when exercising. The underlying causes of such conditions may not be obvious when the horse is examined at rest but may be much easier to see when he is working.

Predictably, a horse may not like having an endoscope pushed up his nose. Many horses will tolerate it with a nose twitch in place, however. With a horse that really objects, a short-acting tranquilizer can usually convince him to cooperate.

Radiographs (X rays)

X *rays* can be very helpful in diagnosing equine respiratory disease in certain areas, such as the head or lungs. Unfortunately, getting good radiographs of the horse's respiratory tract in the field can be a bit of a challenge because the horse is so big and the power put out by portable X-ray units is relatively weak (it takes a lot of X-ray power to get through the chest of a horse). Still, good field X rays can help locate problems in the horse's head, such as bad teeth, or sinuses and guttural pouches filled with discharge, to name a few. However, for most other radiographic examinations, you're going to have to transport your horse to a good clinic where he can be sedated and evaluated with a powerful X-ray machine. And, since hospitals develop the X rays as they are being taken, if the view isn't just right, it's pretty easy to do it again.

Ultrasound

Ultrasound machines use sound waves to produce an image. The sound wave is generated from the machine, enters tissue, and bounces back when it hits body tissues or fluids (it "echoes"). A computer analyzes the echoes to produce a gray-scaled, black-and-white image that can be seen on the ultrasound screen.

Whereas X rays are mainly used for looking at bone and gas, ultrasound is primarily useful for examining soft tissue. Ultrasound probes of differing frequencies can be placed on the horse's head or chest to evaluate swellings or look deep into the horse's body. So, for example, if your horse has a swelling under his jaw, an ultrasound examination might be useful in telling you if there's fluid in the swelling that could be sampled or drained. An ultrasound exam of the chest might tell your veterinarian that there's fluid accumulating there (as happens in cases of shipping fever) or might allow him or her to see an abscess that's developing in the lung (as happens in a young horse with a *Rhodococcus equi* infection). Ultrasound is actually more sensitive than an X ray in determining the character and quality of the chest fluid that can accompany respiratory disease, and the machines are much more portable.

Taking Samples from the Respiratory Tract

There are many reasons why your veterinarian might want to take samples from one or more areas of your horse's respiratory tract. Samples of various areas can help your veterinarian determine the underlying cause of your horse's disease, monitor the horse's response to the disease, and/or see how well your horse is responding to the therapy that has been prescribed.

Many useful samples can be obtained either by direct swabbing or via the endoscope. Sterile swabs can be used to recover material for viral isolation or bacterial culture, or to obtain fluid specimens that can be directly examined for various cells that might give a clue as to the type of, or the response to, disease. In the same vein, fluid samples sucked up with a syringe and sterile pipette from such areas as the guttural pouches can provide valuable clues as to the disease process. However, not all samples can be obtained easily or relatively non-invasively, and so in some cases, the process becomes a bit more involved.

Tracheal Wash

When the horse's air passages are pumping out secretions, or when a disease process prevents the horse's lungs from clearing secretions normally, those secretions can accumulate in the horse's windpipe (his trachea). A *tracheal wash* is one way to collect those secretions, and can be done in one of two ways.

If your veterinarian has a long-enough endoscope and the proper sampling devices, it's possible to get good samples for analysis from an endoscopic exam. However, such scopes tend to be expensive, and not every veterinarian has access to them. So, in many instances, your veterinarian may choose to get a tracheal sample by means of a minor surgical technique.

The surgery involves clipping the hair from your horse's neck, thoroughly cleansing the site, and inserting a large bore needle through the skin into the trachea. Then, a sterile collection catheter is run through the needle down into the trachea. A small volume of sterile saline is pushed in through the catheter and immediately pulled back out—the fluid that's collected is then sent to the lab for bacterial culture and cell analysis.

Although the procedure sounds a bit dramatic, don't worry. The complications from this technique are infrequent and usually quite minor. The horse certainly isn't in any danger of drowning from the small amount of saline used—even if the saline was not sucked back out, the horse's body would rapidly absorb the fluid. Infection of the soft tissue surrounding the needle is possible, but that possibility is minimized by the thorough cleansing, and if it does occur, it can generally be treated easily. Finally, if the catheter is somehow severed inside the horse's trachea or when it's withdrawn, the horse usually coughs and gets rid of the piece of catheter promptly.

Bronchoalveolar Lavage

Bronchoalveolar lavage (BAL) is a means to get fluid and cells from deeper in the horse's air passages. It can be done in the field using a special catheter, with or without the assistance of an endoscope. The BAL tube is passed down the horse's trachea, into the lungs, until it becomes wedged against a bronchus that is the same diameter as the tube. As in the tracheal wash procedure, fluid is pushed through the tube and immediately aspirated, which obtains samples that can be sent to the lab for analysis. BAL is most useful for disease conditions that involve the lungs and is especially helpful in diagnosing airway disease in which there is a lot of inflammation, such as "heaves."

Thoracocentesis (Chest Tap)

Tapping the horse's chest is a relatively easy and uncomplicated way to sample fluid from around his lungs. An ultrasound exam can be very helpful in determining the best spot from which to obtain the fluid and save the horse a few needle pokes. To do a *chest tap*, your veterinarian inserts a short needle or catheter between the horse's ribs and into the chest and fluid is removed. A normal horse has a small amount of clear, yellow fluid between the lungs and the inside of the chest wall, but in some disease conditions—shipping fever, for example—there may be a lot of cloudy fluid that needs not only to be analyzed, but removed.

Lung Biopsies

It is possible to go in through the horse's side and get a piece of lung for examination under the microscope. *Biopsies* can provide both a diagnosis and a prognosis, telling you what the problem is and how likely it is that your horse will recover from it. However, it's not a procedure that is without risk, most particularly that of severe bleeding, even death. Accordingly, most veterinarians don't recommend lung biopsies unless other examination techniques haven't given an answer. It's the rare disease that requires a lung biopsy for diagnosis.

Advanced Imaging Techniques

Nuclear scintigraphy, most commonly used for the evaluation of musculoskeletal problems in the horse, has some application to respiratory disease. For example, scans can detect obscure bone fractures, tooth root abscesses, or bone infection, to name a few. Scintigraphy can also be used to directly study lung function. Of course, such machines require an investment of time and money to utilize properly and are generally only available at private referral hospitals and universities.

In human medicine, *computed tomography (CT)* scans and *magnetic resonance imaging (MRI)* tests are often used in assessing respiratory problems. Unfortunately, these techniques currently have limited usefulness for the horse, for a couple of reasons. First of all, the machines involved are really expensive. Second, they're not well suited for horses—the size of the horse makes it virtually impossible to obtain good images (although they could conceivably be used with foals). Finally, in order to obtain good images of the respiratory tract from these machines, the horse has to be anesthetized, and putting a horse with an already compromised respiratory tract under general anesthesia is a risky proposition.

By using one or more of the preceding techniques, your veterinarian will come up with an approach to treatment. The next chapter discusses what some of those treatments may be.

CHAPTER

3

Medical Treatments

In the course of treating disease of the horse's respiratory tract, you're likely to come across any number of suggested treatments. Of course, the ideal treatment for any condition aims to eliminate the underlying cause. Unfortunately, in some cases, the underlying cause may not be known, or a cure may not be possible.

Frequently, treating disease means that the horse will be given one or more pharmaceutical agents. Appropriately prescribed pharmaceuticals may assist the horse's body in responding to disease and returning to normal. However, pharmaceuticals are not the *only* important consideration, and good medicine is more than just giving drugs. Many respiratory disease conditions have underlying causes that can be recognized and eliminated, preventing further problems. Thus, if possible, you'll want to work closely with your veterinarian—who may elect to use one or more of the diagnostic procedures outlined in the preceding chapter—so that you might be able to uncover the root cause of your horse's problem.

METHODS OF ADMINISTRATION

If a diagnosis of a respiratory disease has been made and the disease is something that is likely to respond to a form of medical treatment, the medication is going to have to get into the horse somehow. There are a variety of drugs and drug formulations, but there are relatively few methods of administration.

Some drugs must be given by *intravenous (IV)* injection. Drugs may be given IV for one of several reasons. Many IV medications are simply too irritating to give by any other means. For example, if you were to put a drug such as *phenylbutazone* ("bute") into the muscle, you'd likely cause a big abscess. However, phenylbutazone can be safely administered directly into the vein, where the large blood volume rapidly dilutes the drug. Intravenous administration of drugs offers some advantages for the horse. Drugs given IV reach higher levels in the bloodstream than by any other route of administration, and they get into the system the fastest. However, although drug levels rise rapidly when given IV, they also fall more rapidly, since the body is more quickly able to start removing the drugs from the system. Of course, IV drugs may be somewhat inconvenient for people who may not feel comfortable giving shots into the horse's vein (a technique that is not without problems). Furthermore, if non-veterinarians give IV injections, certain insurance policies may not be required to pay if something goes wrong with the treatment. Alternative routes of administration may be desirable, particularly for a horse treated at the stable or barn.

Many drugs are given the *intramuscular (IM)* route. IM shots result in lower drug levels (though certainly high enough to be effective) and generally stay in the system for the longest time because the drugs are slowly absorbed from the site where they are given. Unfortunately, as with repeated IV injections, some horses may resent IM administration of drugs—you really can't blame them for disliking getting jabbed with a needle.

Orally administered drugs offer a couple of big advantages in that the medications don't have to be sterile, and horses don't usually kick or strike out when they are given. Given those advantages, it's too bad that many drugs, such as *penicillin*, aren't well absorbed when given orally. Of course, since horses often seem intent on trying to thwart people's best intentions, many horses will not voluntarily eat oral formulations. Consequently, any number of methods to disguise oral drugs are bandied about the barn (molasses, pancake syrup, and Kool-Aid™, to name a few). Some oral medications can be formulated into pastes, which work well in theory. Of course in practice, many horses resent pastes in their mouth. Some will object vigorously to efforts to squirt in a paste and may spit it out (especially if there happens to be any feed in their mouth at the time). Oral formulations may be more convenient, but they're not always easy to give, either.

Drugs may also be given to a horse via aerosol. *Aerosolized drug therapy* has been the standard approach to the treatment of human non-infectious respiratory disease for years. Several devices have been made available that deliver medications directly into the horse's air passages. In general, aerosol delivery systems are one of two types.

Nebulizers use ultrasound or air to generate small particles. Early nebulizers were only marginally effective, mostly because they weren't very efficient at producing particles small enough to get into the horse's air passages. Today, most nebulizers are designed to generate particles that are one to five microns—small enough to get down into the horse's air passages, (assuming that they're not obstructed). Nebulizers can be used with a variety of different medications. As a general rule, ultrasonic nebulizers can get larger volumes of solution into aerosol than can pneumatic (air-driven) nebulizers, and thus may be preferred for things like antibiotic solutions. Ultrasonic nebulizers are much more expensive than pneumatics, however.

There are two concerns about the use of nebulizers, particularly in the field. One is that they are quite happy to draw just about anything that's in the air through them. So, if you're in a dusty environment, a nebulizer may be a good way of getting dust deep down into your horse's lungs. Secondly, if nebulizers are not kept clean, they're very effective at seeding the lower air passages with disease-causing agents.

More recently developed devices allow for the administration of *metered-dose inhaler canisters*, most commonly used for the treatment of people with conditions such as asthma (fig. 5; also see p. 77). There are several advantages to the use of such devices, including rapid delivery of medication (as compared to nebulizers), consistent doses of the administered drug, reduced risk of contamination, and no need for electricity. The drugs are already formulated into small enough particles so that they can get deep into the horse's respiratory tract. By using such equipment, inhalant medications can be given to the horse.

Aerosol administration of drugs offers a couple of distinct advantages. Since the drugs are applied directly to the spot where they're needed, they're very effective. Direct application allows lower drug doses to be used, minimizing side effects. With a little bit of training, horse owners can easily learn to use them. In fact, assuming that the horse tolerates the aerosol system, this method's biggest drawback is its cost.

FIGURE 5

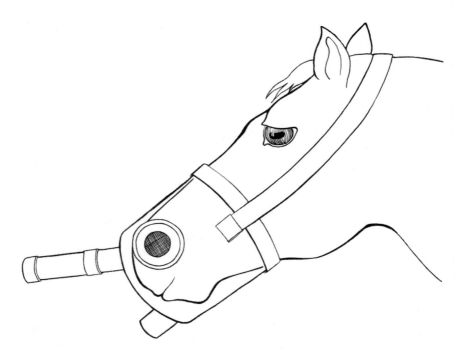

*The horse can be administered inhalant medication
with the Equine Aeromask™.*

Antimicrobials (Antibiotics and Antibacterials)

Antibiotics come from naturally occurring sources, such as mold or plants. *Antibacterials* are substances that are manufactured in the laboratory. Both attempt to kill bacteria. Since their introduction in the mid-twentieth century, such substances have revolutionized the treatment of disease, including respiratory disease.

If your horse contracts an infectious respiratory disease, he may be a candidate for treatment with antimicrobial agents. Under most circumstances, these drugs do not eliminate infection, rather, they kill or control the growth of bacteria until the horse's immune system is able to take charge and clean up the infection. In a horse that is very sick, more than one agent may be used at the same time— using multiple antibiotics that work together helps kill the widest possible range of bacteria.

That said, it's been estimated that something like 70 percent of all infectious diseases will be taken care of by the horse's body without additional help. The problem, of course, is that you can't always tell if your horse is going to be among the 30 percent that aren't so lucky. Thus, in many cases, a horse is treated with antibiotic or antibacterial agents "just in case."

There may be reasons not to use antibiotics and antibacterial agents in treating equine respiratory disease. For example, bacteria do not cause all of the infectious respiratory diseases of the horse. Viruses cause many forms of respiratory disease, and viruses are not susceptible to these drugs. Still, a viral infection is sometimes treated with antibiotics or antibacterials under the rationale that the drugs may help prevent the development of a secondary, bacterial infection. While this sounds good, there's actually little evidence that such secondary infections happen very often.

If antibiotic and antibacterial agents are needed, they should be used at appropriate doses and for an appropriate amount of time. There's good evidence that the indiscriminate use of antibiotic and antibacterial agents creates strains of bacteria that are antibiotic resistant. Bacteria, like everything else, like to live. When constantly exposed to antibiotic or antibacterial drugs, some bacteria are not killed and actually may develop the ability to live in the presence of such drugs and pass on such resistance to other bacteria.

What does this mean? Like most everything else in medicine,

there are rarely black and white answers. If your horse gets a respiratory infection, antibiotics and antibacterials are often a good way to get rid of it. Still, drugs are not benign, and there's no need to give them for every little rise in your horse's temperature or every little dribble of nasal discharge. The selection of the proper antibiotic or antibacterial agent is important, and diagnostic tests, such as attempting to isolate and grow the bacteria to see which antibiotics are most effective (a culture and sensitivity test) may be recommended. Lots of factors help decide what is the most appropriate choice of drug therapy for your horse, and your veterinarian is the best person to make those decisions.

Antibiotics are surprisingly free of side effects, although they do occur. For example, members of the *aminoglycoside* group of antibiotics, such as the commonly used drug *gentamycin*, have the potential to cause kidney problems. The potential for side effects may be increased if a horse is extremely ill. A very sick horse may not metabolize drugs normally, and your veterinarian may find it useful to monitor drug levels in this case. Doses of antibiotic and antibacterial agents may be quite different in foals than in adult horses, and certain drugs may not be appropriate for foals (and vice versa). Some antibiotics are associated with the development of diarrhea. All of these factors point out the importance of using antibiotics and antibacterial agents judiciously and under the direction of your veterinarian.

Non-Steroidal Anti-Inflammatory Drugs (NSAIDs)

Drugs that are *non-steroidal* (they don't have the chemical configuration that is typical of steroid drugs) and *anti-inflammatory* (they help reduce inflammation) are often used in the treatment of equine respiratory disease. There are a number of such drugs available, including *phenylbutazone* or "bute"(the most common), *flunixin meglumine* (Banamine®, known as Finadyne® in the UK), *aspirin*, *ketoprofen* (Ketofen®), and several others.

In the horse's respiratory tract, and particularly in the lungs, uncontrolled inflammation can be very damaging. Even though inflammation is a normal process that helps the horse's body isolate and remove injurious agents and/or injured tissue, the complex series of events that characterize the inflammatory process can result in permanent damage to the horse, particularly in the lungs. Chronic inflammation in the lungs can cause permanent changes in lung tissue and decrease normal respiratory function. Inflammatory cells cause willy-nilly destruction of anything in the inflamed area. Thus, *NSAIDs* are often one of the first treatments suggested by an attending veterinarian.

NSAIDs have other potential benefits, as well. For one, they help control fever. Fever, in and of itself, is not a disease; in a way, a fever is thought to be a "natural" response—an attempt by the horse to make his body less hospitable to invading organisms. However, even though fever is part of the natural course of many infectious diseases, when a horse has a fever, he often won't eat and may act generally depressed. Thus, many veterinarians may choose to try to reduce the fever of a horse with respiratory disease.

In truth, the medical community is somewhat divided about whether most fevers should be controlled (there's little argument that really high fevers should be controlled). Some people feel that it's best to leave most fevers alone and let the disease run its course, hoping that the fever will assist treatment efforts. It is also easier to recognize a favorable response to antibiotic/antibacterial therapy if the fever goes down on its own. In truth, *not* treating a fever can be a bit risky for a veterinarian, unless the veterinarian knows the client well. That's because the veterinarian who does not treat a fever may not be living up to his client's expectations. After all, most people with sick animals want to do something for them. Controlling a fever probably doesn't cause any harm—if it did, it most likely would have been noted a long time ago. It does seem to be agreed that you should either control your horse's fever, or not, and if you're going to control it, you should do so by giving the appropriate drugs at regular intervals and appropriate doses so as to avoid peaks and valleys in your horse's temperature.

Non-steroidal anti-inflammatory drugs also help control pain. Some respiratory conditions, such as *pleuropneumonia*, are very painful. A horse with such a condition may not eat well, or even walk well, due to pain coming from his chest. Consequently, there are some humane reasons for using NSAIDs in the treatment of respiratory disease, though the drugs are just not all *that* potent when it comes to relieving pain. Consider aspirin—if you were really hurting, would you expect aspirin to take all the pain away?

NSAIDs may also be useful in combating the effects of bacterial toxins that may be released from diseased lung tissue, which can occur in severe infection. Such toxins can have all sorts of unwanted secondary effects, including an association with the development of complications, such as *laminitis*.

While it's never a good idea to keep a horse on drugs indefinitely, in general, horses tolerate NSAID therapy rather well. There certainly are occasional complications associated with these drugs—most notably, ulcers of the gastrointestinal tract and kidney problems—but the true incidence of complications appears to be much, much less than the popular concern about them would indicate. NSAIDs are not "horse killers," and they can be an important part of the treatment regimen for a horse with respiratory disease.

Corticosteroids

Corticosteroids are potent inhibitors of inflammation. Currently, they're the most effective drugs available for the relief of inflammation associated with allergic and inflammatory disease of the horse's airways. Among other things, corticosteroids help prevent some of the bad effects of inflammation and help reduce the mucus production that clogs air passages. However, corticosteroids shouldn't generally be used for the treatment of respiratory tract infection because they tend to suppress the horse's immune system.

Corticosteroids have achieved something of an unwarranted reputation as "dangerous" drugs. Some people have tried to associate cortiosteroids with the development of laminitis. Although such an association has never been proven, it's always prudent to use such drugs in the lowest dose possible, for the shortest time possible, so as to prevent side effects (just as you should with any drug). Fortunately, the advent of aerosol-delivered corticosteroids has allowed administration of these drugs in a manner that is both safer and more effective.

Bronchodilators

Drugs that dilate the horse's air passages have many uses in the treatment of equine respiratory disease. By opening the airways, drugs such as *clenbuterol* or *albuterol* help the horse breathe with less effort. They don't get at the root cause of disease, but because of their fast action, they can be very helpful at relieving clinical signs of respiratory distress. Like corticosteroids, *bronchodilating agents* can be given either orally or via aerosols.

Antihistamines

Histamine is a potent chemical that is normally found in the horse's body. It has a wide variety of effects on various body tissues of the horse, including blood vessels and the muscles of the horse's bronchi. Histamine is also one of the chemical substances released during *allergic hypersensitivity reactions*. Because of the involvement of histamine in allergic reactions, *antihistamines*—drugs that block the effect of histamine—have commonly been prescribed for the treatment of allergic respiratory disease in the horse. Unfortunately, there are a number of different body chemicals involved in allergic-type reactions, and perhaps because of this, antihistamines have not been shown to be of much use for their control.

Expectorant and Mucolytic Agents

Sometimes drugs are given to a horse to increase (*expectorants*) or loosen (*mucolytics*) secretions from the lungs. Bronchodilators, such as clenbuterol, may perform such a function; so do substances such as *potassium iodide*, given intravenously, or *N-acetylcysteine*, which is usually given via a nebulizer. Some people have advocated giving large amounts of intravenous saline solution, particularly to a horse with allergic airway disease, in an effort to loosen mucus. This is something that should only be done under veterinary supervision.

Cough Suppressants

Many products are available that attempt to suppress the cough that is often associated with equine respiratory disease. They are rarely useful and there's little evidence that they work anyway. Cough is actually a very important body mechanism to help remove secretions from the respiratory tract, and suppressing such a mechanism is rarely a good idea. If you treat the underlying cause, the cough will go away, as well.

Immune System Modulators

One novel approach to treating respiratory disease in the horse involves the use of substances intended to affect the horse's immune system. *Immunostimulants* are intended to activate immune cells, mostly to assist in the treatment of infection. The effectiveness of such drugs is pretty much unknown and may also depend, to some extent, on the efficiency of the immune system of an individual animal. Immune system stimulants come from a variety of sources, including bacterial cell-wall fractions, inactivated bacteria, sterile purified goat serum, the antiparasitic agent *levamisole*, and *interferon*—a product developed in humans to help fight off viral infection. Still, it's pretty hard to know what to say about such products, given that there hasn't yet been good clinical investigation, and so there's a resulting lack of knowledge about the benefits or potential side effects. As veterinary immunology develops and interaction between the immune system and disease agents is better understood, immune system modulators may be used more effectively and without adverse effects on the horse.

"Alternative" Treatments

Treatments called "alternative" or "complementary" have been heavily promoted in veterinary medicine over the past decade or so. Whether it is because such treatments are "natural," represent the wisdom of ancient cultures, or affect vital energies, horse owners may be tempted to employ them because of a desire to do everything that they can to help their horses.

While such underlying desires may certainly be understandable, in fact, such treatments have not been shown to have any effect at all in horses—or even people. For example, acupuncture, chiropractic, and homeopathy have not been shown to help people with asthma or bronchitis. Although such treatments may be recommended for a horse with allergic airway disease ("heaves"), given their lack of usefulness in people, there's little reason to think that they might help a horse. Similarly, although plants certainly may contain substances that have pharmacologic activity, no plants have been shown to be useful in the treatment of equine respiratory disease of any form. Add in the documented problems with contamination, lack of purity, and lack of content regulation for such products, and there's ample additional reason to view them with skepticism. Dabbling with such treatments in cases of infectious respiratory disease, particularly if they are used instead of proven-effective therapies, may be dangerous.

These interventions seem to serve mostly to make people feel good about trying to help horses, but such feelings come at a financial cost. You're much more likely to help your horse's respiratory problem—and save money in the process—by using proven-effective therapies at the direction of your veterinarian.

Upper Airway Problems

The upper airway of the horse is made up of all of the parts that lead to the windpipe, from the nostrils to the larynx. Just about any structure in the upper airway can be affected by some sort of medical problem, but there are a few that deserve special attention.

NASAL PASSAGE PROBLEMS

The horse's nasal passages are not a big source of trouble. In older horses, cancer of the nasal passage can occasionally be seen (and are generally very difficult to treat successfully). However, in some adult horses, a slow-growing, non-cancerous mass can start from the ethmoturbinate bones at the end of the passages. Untreated, the masses can take up space in the nasal passages, grow into the pharynx, or spread into the sinuses. No one knows why they occur. The masses are called *ethmoid hematomas*.

Most commonly, ethmoid hematomas cause a bloody discharge from the affected nasal passage (but so do other growths). If they get large enough, they can obstruct the passage, causing breathing noises and difficulties. Other signs include coughing, head shaking, bad breath, and, in severe cases, facial deformities. The diagnosis is usually confirmed with an endoscope. A biopsy can help distinguish between a cancerous and non-cancerous growth.

Veterinarians try to treat ethmoid hematomas by destroying them. A number of methods have been tried, including several surgical techniques—even laser surgery. Chemical destruction of the mass by direct injection of *formaldehyde* has also been tried. Regardless of the approach, however, these growths can be very difficult to cure. Even though they are not considered malignant (they don't spread through the horse's body, ethmoid hematomas tend to regrow, much like cancerous tumors.

SINUS PROBLEMS

Sinus problems can be a real pain to diagnose and treat in the horse because the sinuses are large, their anatomy is intricate, and they're hard to access. Most sinus diseases cause a snotty nose, with the discharge coming from the nostril that's on the same side as the affected sinus. Sinus disease can also cause breathing noises, swelling about the face, or even tearing, if the tear duct that runs from the eye to the nostril is compressed. Sinus disease can be primary, that is, the problem is with the sinus itself, or, quite commonly, secondary to infections of the roots of the upper cheek teeth.

Percussion, or tapping on the horse's skull, can occasionally be used to diagnose sinus problems. One sinus is tapped with the fingers, and then the other, and the veterinarian listens for differences in the sound. Percussion can be a bit tricky, however, and either endoscopy or an X ray are generally needed to help confirm a clinical diagnosis.

It's also possible to go directly into a horse's sinus while the horse is standing. While pretty dramatic-looking, it's actually quite safe and not all that difficult (once you know how to do it). A large bore needle or steel pin can be placed directly through the bone, into the sinus, and fluid can be sucked out for analysis. Sterile fluids can also be flushed into the hole to rinse out infected material. In some cases, the hole can be made large enough to allow the veterinarian to put an endoscope into the sinus and look around. All while the horse is standing under mild sedation: amazing!

Treatment of sinus infection involves rinsing out the sinuses on a regular basis, usually accompanied by systemic antibiotic treatment. If a tooth is the problem, the offending tooth may need to be removed. Odd things that occur in sinuses, such as the occasional tumor seen mostly in older horses, or fungal infections, may require special treatment, or may not be treatable at all.

GUTTURAL POUCH PROBLEMS

Occasionally, one or both of the guttural pouches that open into the horse's pharynx can become problematic. While not common, *guttural pouch disease* can be a bit tricky to treat, mostly because the guttural pouch is an air-filled sac that doesn't have any small blood vessels weaving through it. This makes it difficult to get therapeutic levels of drugs into it using the most common routes of administration.

Empyema

Empyema means that a body cavity is full of pus—the thick, whitish liquid product of inflammation made of white blood cells and debris. Pus occurs as a result of the body's attempt to fight off disease. A horse with empyema of his guttural pouch or pouches is usually examined because of discharge coming from one or both of the nostrils. Other signs of guttural pouch empyema include coughing, difficulty swallowing, or swelling in the throat. The diagnosis can be confirmed by direct endoscopic examination, or by X rays, which may show that there's fluid in the pouch.

Treating empyema of the guttural pouch can be challenging; it involves draining and rinsing out the pouch. This can be done daily, or your veterinarian may also elect to put a tube (a catheter) into the pouch and leave it there for a few days. The pouch is flushed, usually with non-irritating saline solutions, until it runs clear. In some cases, the pus can dry up and form hard little rocks called *chondroids*, which may need to be removed surgically. How helpful systemic antibiotics are is a bit of a guess, since they have difficulty reaching the pouch. It's pretty much a given that antibiotics alone won't do the trick.

Tympany

Tympany is a condition found in young foals, in which air gets trapped in the guttural pouch or pouches. This causes the throat area to blow up like a balloon and also causes cough, breathing noises, and difficulty in swallowing. Percussion of the air-filled area will reveal a hollow sound, much like thumping on a soccer ball. Endoscopy and/or X rays can also be used to confirm the diagnosis. Sometimes, tympany is complicated by infection, so it's important to look for both.

The cause of guttural pouch tympany is usually improper development of the opening into the pouch, which causes it to act as a one-way valve. Air gets in but doesn't get out, and as a result, the pouch blows up like a balloon. In some young horses, air may accumulate due to a problem with the nervous system. Regardless, successful treatment usually involves surgery to enlarge the opening in one or both pouches to let the air out.

Mycosis

Some horses develop a fungal infection in one or both of their guttural pouches. These infections can be particularly nasty. The first sign may be a bloody nose, which can be extremely serious—even fatal. The fungi often set up shop on one or more of the big arteries that pass through the pouch, and when the fungi eat through the artery, massive bleeds can occur.

Treatment of guttural pouch mycosis generally involves surgery. Medical treatment alone is generally tedious and long-term, and it doesn't always work. And, when medical therapy doesn't work, the outcome is often fatal. Surgery is recommended to tie-off the affected artery so that it can't bleed if it's ruptured. Surgical treatment is generally successful but presents many technical challenges to the surgeon, and failures do occur.

PHARYNGEAL PROBLEMS

Problems with the pharynx can occur in horses of any age. For example, a foal can be born with a *cleft palate*, which is most commonly noted when the nursing foal is seen with milk draining out of his nostrils (the milk comes through a split in the hard palate back out through the nostrils). This, and other rare conditions that can be seen in newborns, such as inadequate development of the pharynx, may require surgical treatment. Surgical treatment is very difficult and, at best, only partially successful. Thankfully, these conditions are so unusual that it's unlikely that most horse owners (or veterinarians) will ever see a case.

Trauma to the pharynx can affect horses of any age and can be caused by penetrating wounds, stomach tubes, or blows to the throat area, to name a few. Stomach tubes, sometimes used by veterinarians to get medication into a horse with a condition such as colic, or tracheal tubes used during general anesthesia, can bruise the pharyngeal region. Signs of pharyngeal trauma include difficulty swallowing and abnormal breathing noises. Your veterinarian may want to use endoscopes or X rays to come up with a diagnosis. Depending on the underlying cause, treatments will vary, as well.

When horses get to be adults, the most common problems of the pharynx affect performance. One of the more common conditions is called *dorsal displacement of the soft palate*. The soft palate, which normally fits over the larynx in its "button hole" configuration, will displace upwards—"unbuttoning", as it were—and cause breathing noises and poor performance. Unfortunately, trying to figure out the reason this happens can be a bit frustrating, and because the cause can be so elusive, finding a successful treatment can be difficult. One common treatment is to use a "tongue-tie"—a leather strap or a bandana, for example—to tie the horse's tongue to the jaw (fig. 6). This helps keep the horse from swallowing and the palate from unbuttoning as it normally does when the horse swallows. If this technique doesn't help, various surgical solutions may be proposed. Unfortunately, none of the currently used surgical treatments for this problem are consistently successful, but newer treatments, such as a surgical approach to pull the larynx forward, will hopefully be more promising.

Pharynxes can become inflamed, too. Inflammation of the pharynx probably occurs due to the variety of viruses, mold, dust, and bacteria that the horse can inhale, particularly while stabled. In this condition, called *lymphoid hyperplasia*, little bumps appear on the walls of the pharynx because the inhaled material stimulates the lymphatic system, which is full of immune cells (hyperplasia means there is an abnormal increase in the number of normal cells in a tissue). These little bumps contain *lymphoid tissue*, which is always present and acts as the horse's equivalent to a person's tonsils. It's been well demonstrated that the condition occurs mostly in young horses, just as tonsillitis occurs mostly in young people.

Some people have tried to correlate lymphoid hyperplasia with poor performance. Most veterinarians, however, seem to think that it's a condition that has little, if any, affect on a horse's athletic ability (unless the condition is severe). Veterinarians may elect to treat severe cases a number of ways, including spraying anti-inflammatory solutions right into the pharynx.

LARYNGEAL PROBLEMS
Laryngeal problems typically interrupt normal airflow and cause signs of decreased performance and/or respiratory noise. Problems with the larynx are most commonly seen in adult horses. While most laryngeal problems may be primary—that is, the problem is localized in the larynx—they can also be secondary to such conditions as *hyperkalemic periodic paralysis*, a genetic condition affecting Quarter Horses of the "Impressive" line (this condition is an excep-

FIGURE 6

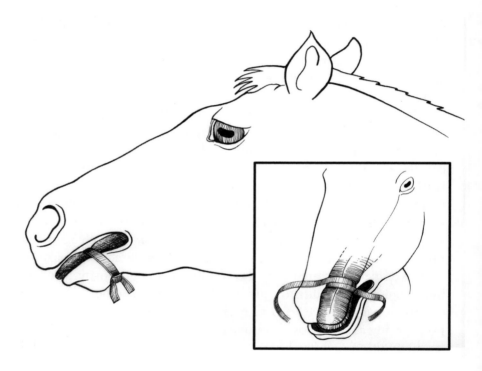

A *"tongue-tie" is often used to treat dorsal
displacement of the soft palate.*

tion in that it usually affects very young foals). As a rule, the various conditions that affect the horse's larynx are diagnosed with an endoscope and often require surgical treatment.

Without doubt, the most commonly seen laryngeal problem is a partial or complete paralysis of the left cartilage that guards the horse's trachea. The condition is called *left laryngeal hemiplegia*, and it has been recognized for at least 200 years. It can be seen in horses of all breeds and occupations and is most commonly diagnosed when horses are young, after they first start to work hard. Most horses with laryngeal paralysis make abnormal, loud, exercise-related, respiratory sounds—commonly referred to as "roaring"—and a significant number of them don't tolerate strenuous exercise well due to breathing difficulties. Laryngeal paralysis—which can also very occasionally affect the right cartilage, or sometimes even both—affects the horse's performance because it narrows the air passage, and the horse breathes in less air than he normally would.

You can see the cartilage using an endoscope. When a horse has a paralysis of the left cartilage, it hangs limply in the airway. It doesn't pull back when the horse breathes, as it normally would. Instead, when the horse needs to breathe rapidly during exercise, the cartilage flaps in the breeze of the incoming air. This causes noise—the limp cartilage acts just like the paper membrane in a kazoo—and gives rise to a common name for the laryngeal cartilage, the "flapper."

In laryngeal paralysis, the muscles to the cartilage don't function properly because of problems with the nerve that activates them. The nerve problem can have any number of causes and can occur with many other diseases. For example, both upper and lower respiratory tract disease are associated with paralysis of the left cartilage. Paralysis of both cartilages has been seen with liver disease or following general anesthesia. It's also been seen in association with fungal infection of the guttural pouch.

While the origin of the problem is unknown in many cases, in others, nerve damage occurs when irritating substances—such as many commonly used pharmaceuticals—are accidentally injected outside of the horse's jugular vein. The nerve, which runs right alongside the jugular vein, can be damaged by the inflammation and scarring that can result from misplaced injections. This is one good reason your veterinarian should give intravenous injections.

Most often, laryngeal hemiplegia is corrected by surgery that "ties back" the affected cartilage. The surgeon places one or two large sutures into the cartilage and ties them tightly, opening up the horse's airway in the process. Of course, the surgery causes its own complications, such as coughing and difficulty swallowing. Furthermore, not every horse that makes a noise due to laryngeal paralysis needs surgery. In fact, horses that aren't elite athletes can do just fine, although they'll make a noise if they're asked to run hard. Essentially, surgery should be carefully discussed with the surgeon prior to making a decision.

One or both of the laryngeal cartilages can become inflamed or infected, as well. A horse with this condition typically shows up with swelling in the throat and may have a hard time breathing. While antibiotics and anti-inflammatory drugs may help resolve some of these cases, chronic cases, or cases that have been resolved but have left significant scarring or malformation of the cartilages, may need surgical treatment. In some severe instances, surgery may be needed to allow the horse to breathe well enough just to stay alive. Unfortunately, the surgery is technically demanding and the outlook for a successful recovery is variable to the extreme, depending on the extent of the disease and how long it's been going on.

Although it's not common, the epiglottis occasionally causes performance horses some problems, as well. The epiglottis can get trapped in the folds of tissue that lie underneath it. If this occurs—and it can only be diagnosed with an endoscope—surgical correction by cutting the entrapping tissue is the usual treatment. Unfortunately, sometimes this problem occurs because the epiglottis is underdeveloped and way too small. In these cases, even when the tissue is removed, the epiglottis may not be able to effectively keep the soft palate "buttoned down" and the horse may still make noise at work.

Lower Airway Problems

In general, when the term "lower airway" is used, it refers to the structures in the horse's chest, most often the horse's lungs (fig. 7). Of particular concern is *pneumonia*, a familiar word defined as inflammation of the lungs with thickening and hardening of the lung tissue. Lung problems are very common in horses of all ages, breeds, and occupations, but each age group has some problems that are peculiar to it.

PROBLEMS OF THE NEWBORN FOAL

Making the move from inside the mare to outside on the ground is a big deal. New babies have to immediately open up their lungs and absorb the fluid that they've been bathing in for the preceding eleven months, all in a very short time. Of course, in most neonates, this transition is seamless. However, poor lung development, infection, or abnormality in the placental connections between mother and baby, among other things, can cause the new foal to get off to a rough start.

Babies breathe rapidly during the first hour that they're alive, with their respiratory rate falling to 30 to 40 breaths per minute after a few hours. The rapid breathing helps to clear the lungs and get oxygen into the foal's body. Problems with the lungs of a new foal can occur due to a variety of conditions, including infection of the placenta or uterus, breathing in *meconium*—the dark "first poop" that's in the foal's intestines, made up of a mixture of various body secretions—or primary lung disease. Such conditions can result in low blood oxygen levels (*hypoxemia*). Problem foals are generally easy to recognize: they may be dull and listless, fail to suckle, or run a fever. When a newborn foal isn't getting enough oxygen, it often means that intensive care treatments such as

FIGURE 7

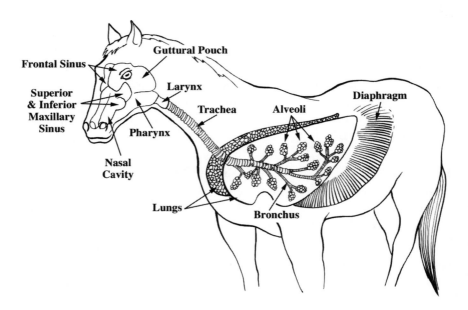

The structures of the upper and lower airways of the horse.

intranasal oxygen therapy will be required. This is best delivered in an appropriate referral hospital setting.

Fortunately, most newborn foals don't have immediate problems. For normal babies, doing everything that you can to prevent respiratory or other health problems is the key to a good start. In that regard, it's absolutely critical to make sure that they drink plenty of the mare's first milk, the *colostrum*, in the first twenty-four hours of their lives. The newborn foal has never been exposed to the world outside. He isn't ready to fight off disease, as he hasn't had time to develop immunity to any disease-causing agents. Colostrum contains the immune factors necessary to help the foal fight off such agents, but they are absorbed through the foal's intestines for about a day only. You can help your new foal get off to a good start by making sure that he's up and suckling vigorously and often. The day after he is born, you can have your veterinarian check his blood to make sure that the absorption of the immune factors found in the colostrum is adequate. If it hasn't been adequate, or if the foal is showing signs of disease, your veterinarian may recommend treatments, such as intravenous infusion of blood plasma from another horse to help booster the foal's immune system.

In new babies, pneumonia is a problem that's seen all too often. There are numerous causes; for example, many different bacteria can cause pneumonia, and for that reason, antibiotics are often cornerstones of treatment. However, pneumonia may be just the tip of the disease iceberg for an affected foal, as it frequently occurs along with infection in other parts of the foal's body. You can't just look at the foal's lungs and forget that they're attached to a foal!

Foals can have trouble breathing for reasons unrelated to infection, too. For example, rib fractures occur in a small percentage of foals. These babies often don't breathe at a normal rate, rather, their breaths are quick and shallow, but it's because their chest hurts, not because they're sick. Severe rib fractures may need to be repaired at a referral facility, but most foals with rib fractures recover uneventfully at home with rest and confinement for a few weeks.

SUCKLING AND WEANING PROBLEMS

Even after a baby gets through the difficult time transitioning to life outside of the mare, respiratory disease looms as a potential problem. In fact, one study, conducted in Texas, showed that respiratory disease was the number one cause of health problems in horses from one to six months of age.

While life with "Mom" is generally good, eventually foals, like all babies, have to grow up and take care of things on their own. In particular, the young horse's immune system has to learn to fend for itself. While the mare's colostrum provides immediate immune protection for the baby horse, that immunity wanes and must be replaced by the foal's own functioning system. During the time when the immunity from the colostrum is waning and the foal's system is getting going, the foal can be particularly susceptible to respiratory disease.

Environmental factors also make the young horse susceptible to the development and spread of respiratory disease. Often, babies are kept crowded together with other babies; much like elementary school for children, it's an ideal way for disease to develop and spread. Add in stresses such as handling, weaning, and, in some areas, preparing for sale, and you've got a situation where the young horse's body is further taxed, making him even more susceptible to disease.

Bacterial Respiratory Disease

Several strains of dangerous bacteria, including *Streptococcus zooepidemicus, Rhodococcus equi,* and *Streptococcus equi* (or "strangles"—see chapter 7), can make a young horse sick with bacterial pneumonia. A young horse with pneumonia may show signs of fever, loss of appetite, cough, increased respiratory rate, and nasal discharge. When your veterinarian listens to the lungs of one of these sick little guys, he will most likely hear all sorts of crackling and wheezing from the gummed-up air passages, unless the disease is quite advanced and the lung tissue is filled with fluid, in which case he may hear nothing much all. Blood samples can help your veterinarian determine how bad the problem really is, and bacterial cultures may be helpful to identify the organism that's causing the problem and to select appropriate antibacterial treatment.

Imaging the lungs of an affected young horse may be very helpful. Lung X rays may help your veterinarian determine the extent of the disease. Normal foal lungs look pretty black on X rays, but if lung tissue becomes hardened and thickened, or the chest cavity starts to fill with fluid, white blotchy areas or a line of fluid may be seen. (Normally, X rays pass right through the air-filled lungs onto the X-ray film, and as a result, lung X rays are black; fluid will stop some of the X rays, so the X-ray film looks whiter when there's fluid in the chest.) Lung abscesses can also be picked up on X rays. An ultrasound examination of the chest cavity may also be helpful.

A particularly problematic bacterial cause of respiratory disease in the young horse is *Rhodococcus equi*. *R. equi* is a bacteria that lives in the ground—even in ground that's never been lived on by horses. This disease can be particularly horrible, as it can cause widespread abscesses in the lung tissue. And, although *R. equi* starts out pretty much like every other respiratory disease, it can involve other tissue, particularly that of the gastrointestinal tract. So, in a horse with a long-established *R. equi* infection, weight loss can be an obvious feature of the disease.

R. equi infections are a big problem in some areas and not a problem at all in others. No one is really sure why this is, but several things might be considered, including the environment (ideal conditions for *R. equi* are warm and dry), how the farm or ranch is managed, and the fact that some strains of the bacteria are better at causing disease than others. However, even on farms at which the disease tends to be a problem, adult horses seem to have an established immunity to the bacteria.

If a diagnosis of *R. equi* is made, usually through a combination of exam findings and bacterial cultures, aggressive treatment is warranted. Identification of the bacteria is particularly important in *R. equi* infection because it is sensitive to antibiotics, such as *erythromycin*, *rifampin*, and *azithromycin*, that aren't typically used for other forms of respiratory disease. Affected animals usually need to be treated for many weeks.

Of course, "an ounce of prevention is worth a pound of cure," and instituting good management procedures is very important for the control of *R. equi* (as well as all respiratory disease). Good management includes avoiding overcrowding, keeping dirt down (so as to avoid putting infective particles into the air), keeping stables clean and well ventilated, and isolating infected animals to keep disease from spreading. Giving foals intravenous doses of blood plasma rich in immune factors against the bacteria has become a foundation of prevention programs on some farms that have chronic problems with *R. equi*; in some circumstances, it may be recommended to give foals one liter of plasma within a week after birth, and then again a few weeks later. Screening foals with blood tests to check for increases in white blood cells may also be of some use.

Viral Respiratory Disease

Much as they can in people, viruses can wreak havoc in the lungs of young horses. Outbreaks of viral respiratory disease can occur at any time of the year but are particularly problematic when young horses are gathered during weaning, showing, and sales. Putting lots of young horses together, particularly in crowded and poorly ventilated conditions, makes it easier for disease to spread, mostly because under such conditions, sick horses easily come into contact with healthy ones. In addition, the stress caused by such concentration can depress the young horse's immune system and make him less able to fight off disease.

Viral respiratory disease looks and acts very much like bacterial respiratory disease, at least in the initial stages, and affected animals develop coughs, fevers, snotty noses, and the other common signs of respiratory disease. Your veterinarian may elect to do any number of diagnostic tests, including blood work, or in severe outbreaks, he or she may attempt to isolate and identify the virus in an effort to control the disease.

Viruses aren't affected by antibiotics so antibiotic therapy won't help a horse with viral respiratory disease. However, it is possible for a bacterial infection to follow one caused by a virus, so your veterinarian may elect to put a young horse with a viral infection on antibiotics, just to be on the safe side. Non-steroidal anti-inflammatory drugs, such as *phenylbutazone* and *flunixin meglumine*, may also be used to help lower fevers and get a young horse to eat, however, they are not without bad side effects—particularly stomach ulcers—and as a result, they should be used wisely and under your veterinarian's direction. It's also helpful to keep a sick young horse isolated, and in a clean, well-ventilated environment for as long as three or four weeks, until he is well and has stopped shedding virus particles. Your veterinarian may suggest as much as one week of rest for every day of fever to give the lungs time to fully heal.

Vaccines are available to help prevent most of the common viral respiratory diseases, such as *influenza* and *rhinopneumonitis*. These can be administered either by intramuscular injection or by intranasal spray. It's now been recognized that the young horse doesn't respond well to vaccines prior to about six months of age, so it doesn't make much sense to vaccinate before then. In addition, the current data would suggest that the intranasal vaccines are somewhat more effective than are the intramuscular vaccines, though, with new vaccines emerging and existing vaccines being subjected to testing, your veterinarian will be able to make appropriate recommendations for your situation. Many veterinarians advise vaccinating broodmares a month or so before foaling in an effort to boost the immune factors in the colostrum. However, while vaccination is important, it's certainly not a substitute for good management. Preventing viral respiratory disease includes such important considerations as reducing stress and isolating new arrivals to a farm for several weeks prior to introducing them to the general population.

ADULT HORSE PROBLEMS

The more common adult lower airway problems, such as shipping fever, heaves, and bleeding from the lungs, deserve special attention, and are subjects of the chapters that follow. However, adult horses—like horses of all ages—also get pneumonia. Proper diagnosis of adult horse pneumonia is similar to that of horses of other ages, involving a combination of clinical and laboratory diagnostic techniques for a number of different viruses and bacteria. Treatment also follows the same general guidelines as those used in horses of other ages, keyed by the selection of appropriate pharmaceuticals to kill bacteria, control fever, and ease breathing. Adult horse pneumonia can be very difficult to take care of and are often complicated by *pleuritis* (see chapter 6)—it may take many weeks of medication for a successful resolution.

Prevention of adult horse lower respiratory disease is best achieved with good management practices and appropriate vaccination schedules constructed with the assistance of your veterinarian. In particular, a number of vaccines exist for the control of the equine influenza virus, with recommended intervals varying from three to twelve months. Some people elect to vaccinate horses in the face of disease outbreaks, but this practice isn't likely to be very effective, since most horses in an outbreak have already been exposed by the time that vaccination is considered. Fortunately, once a horse has had a viral respiratory disease, he usually develops a long-term immunity to future infection.

Pneumothorax is an infrequent condition that occurs when air enters the chest cavity and impairs normal lung function by playing havoc with the negative chest pressure that keeps the lungs inflated and lets the horse breathe normally. Pneumothorax can occur on its own (particularly in a horse that is working at maximum exercise) or as a result of trauma to the chest cavity, such as a penetrating wound. A horse with air in his chest has difficulty breathing, breathes rapidly, or in severe cases, may not be able to get adequate amounts of oxygen into his bloodstream, resulting in blue mucous membranes. This is a serious condition that requires removal of the air from the chest cavity by suction, usually in a hospital setting.

Hernias of the diaphragm—the large muscle that separates the chest cavity from the abdominal cavity—can occur in the horse after trauma. For example, after foaling, a mare may develop a hernia due to the heavy exertion needed to push out the baby. A horse with a diaphragmatic hernia can be tricky to diagnose, as although most will display evidence of respiratory distress, some don't. In fact, some horses with diaphragmatic hernias don't have any clinical signs that would normally be associated with respiratory disease! In particular, a horse with a hole in his diaphragm may colic when the intestines migrate up into the chest cavity. An ultrasound or X ray usually makes a diagnosis (they usually show guts in the chest). It may be possible to correct some of these cases in surgery, but curiously, some horses have long-standing hernias and show few signs of distress. Obviously, proper treatment for each individual horse involves the strict attention of a veterinarian.

There are some rather uncommon problems of adult-horse lower airways to consider, as well. Though very uncommon, cancer can appear in a horse's lungs, either as primary tumors or from cancer of other areas. Lung cancer is essentially impossible to treat successfully, although heroic surgical efforts have reportedly cured at least one case.

6

Pleuropneumonia ("Shipping Fever")

One of the more difficult diseases to affect the horse is *pleuropneumonia*. It's most commonly recognized as "shipping fever" or "travel sickness" because of its association with equine transport. Although pleuropneumonia can certainly affect a horse that hasn't been moved about and can occur as a complication from many forms of respiratory disease, it's association with travel, and the necessity of transporting horses for competition and sales, makes this disease a concern for many horse owners. Fortunately, many of the reasons that this disease occurs are now understood.

Which horses get pleuropneumonia?

Pleuropneumonia doesn't appear to be selective about the age or the sex of the horse it strikes. Thoroughbreds seem to get the disease more often than other horses, but this might be due to any number of other factors, such as they may be transported more often than any other breed. However, in almost every case, some sort of an unusual event in the horse's life—some sort of severe stress—precedes pleuropneumonia.

Transportation is a definite risk factor for development of the disease. That's why, when pleuropneumonia occurs after shipping, the disease is so-commonly called "shipping fever." A horse that is moved frequently about to races or shows is definitely more likely to get pleuropneumonia, and the greater the distance, the greater the risk—a horse transported over 500 miles is more likely to develop the disease than one transported for shorter distances. Transport also keeps the horse in a box full of dust, bacteria, and mold, things that may cause disease in their own right.

What causes pleuropneumonia?

Pleuropneumonia is largely a bacterial disease. It can be caused by any number of bacteria, most of which already live in the horse. Stress in any form seems to be a consistent factor that leads to the development of the disease. Many different things, besides transport, can stress a horse, including food and/or water deprivation, or frequent and intense training. In fact, it's been shown that the function of the defense mechanisms of the lungs, necessary to fight off disease-causing organisms, is impaired by stress. A stressed horse is less able to fight off an infection than unstressed stablemates.

The existence of other medical conditions can make a horse a candidate for pleuropneumonia. For example, viral infection interferes with normal lung function, and a horse that has had a recent viral infection appears to be at risk for developing the disease. Or, a horse with EIPH (discussed in chapter 9) may have areas of damaged lung that are more easily infected, leading to disease. But it's not just respiratory conditions that are a problem—horses that are sick from any number of other diseases can get pleuropneumonia, too. Even surgery can cause enough stress on a horse's system to lead to later development of the disease.

A horse can breathe bacteria and contaminants into his lungs following episodes of *choke*, where feed material gets packed into the esophagus, making it impossible for it to get down to the stomach. In such cases, saliva, feed, and bacteria come running out the horse's nasal passages. If the horse breathes these things into his lungs, pleuropneumonia can result. Occasionally, serious pleuropneumonia can result from foreign material, such as light mineral oil, being introduced into the horse's lungs via a nasogastric tube placed into the trachea instead of the esophagus; that's why veterinarians are very careful that tubes are placed properly before pumping any medication down them.

It has been rather nicely shown that the bacteria that cause "travel sickness" are part of the normal bacteria that live in the horse's pharynx. These bacteria gain access to the lungs, at least in part, because of the head-up posture that the horse is often forced to maintain during travel. When a horse is forced to keep his head up for long periods of time, it favors the movement of the bacteria toward the lungs and makes it harder for the horse to clear the bacteria away—the bacteria can't be moved up the trachea (against gravity) very easily. The longer a horse is kept restrained with his head up, the greater the chance that pleuropneumonia will occur.

Studies have shown that a horse requires six to eight hours where he can lower his head to clear the secretions that accumulate in his air passages. So, unfortunately, making a quick stop on a long trailer ride so that the horse can get out and lower his head is simply not enough. Furthermore, it's not just the actual travel time that should be considered when transporting a horse, but all the extra time, as well, such as waiting to get on and off trailers or airplanes, and road transport to and from airports. It's important to try to keep the time involved with these things to a minimum.

Other factors are also very important. Dehydration, dusty conditions in the hauling vehicle, and unique contaminants, such as exhaust fumes and particulate matter in the air, stress the horse's immune system. Strenuous exercise immediately after transport can also add to the stress—it's a good idea to give a horse some time to rest after a long trip.

What's happening in the horse's chest?

When bacteria gain entry to the horse's lungs and the defense mechanisms aren't successful in removing them, the bacteria begin to grow inside the lungs. As the bacteria grow, they cause damage and inflammation to the lung tissue and inflammation in the air passages, as well. As the disease progresses, the damage and inflammation eventually lead to permanent changes in the lung tissue (the "pneumonia" of pleuropneumonia).

The "pleuro" part of pleuropneumonia comes into play when the bacteria gain access to the outer surfaces of the lung and come in contact with the pleural lining of the inside of the chest. This causes even more inflammation, and the lining—which, if laid out like a blanket, is larger than any blanket you'll ever see—produces fluid. This is called *pleuritis*. Inflammation of any body structure causes discomfort, and inflammation of a large surface such as the pleura of the lungs can make the horse reluctant to walk, eat, or even breathe.

What are the signs of pleuropneumonia?

It's important to be vigilant if your horse is at risk for developing pleuropneumonia. Probably the two most important tools for recognizing that a problem is developing are a handler who's paying attention to, or is familiar with the horse and a thermometer. If an at-risk horse is not eating, drinking, or acting normally, or starts to develop a fever, it's important to recognize such signs immediately so that treatment can be started—and the offending stress stopped—as soon as possible.

Once it becomes established, pleuropneumonia is not necessarily easy to diagnose. Indeed, horses are referred to hospitals for pleuropneumonia for any number of reasons, including weight loss, recurring fever, colic, laminitis, muscle stiffness, and chronic cough. The most common sign of the disease is rapid breathing—a horse with pleuropneumonia often takes quick, shallow breaths, probably because his chest hurts from the infection inside. He may walk stiffly and slowly, as well (one reason why the disease can be confusing).

Once your veterinarian starts listening to the horse's chest, he may hear many different sounds, from crackles and rubbing sounds, to muffled sounds, to nothing at all (when fluid accumulates in the chest cavity, it is harder to hear sounds). Ultrasound examination is very useful for finding fluid lines and evaluating the severity of the underlying disease in the horse's lungs. Chest taps—sometimes obtained with ultrasound guidance—can provide samples of the fluid for analysis, as well as for trying to culture the organisms that are causing the disease.

Other signs may be helpful in coming up with a diagnosis of pleuropneumonia. Fever is a common sign in early cases, but may be less consistent once the disease gets established. An affected horse may cough or have nasal discharge. Some horses even get swelling along their belly, chest, or (in male horses) sheath. Nevertheless, a diagnosis of pleuropneumonia is not one that's necessarily easily achieved.

How is pleuropneumonia treated?

The cornerstone of therapy for pleuropneumonia is antimicrobial therapy. Usually, "broad spectrum" combinations of antimicrobials are used, targeted at different types of bacteria, including those anaerobic bacteria that can live without any oxygen. Anti-inflammatory drugs may help reduce the pain of the disease and may help encourage the horse to eat. In severely debilitated cases, providing the horse with additional fluids may also be required.

When fluid accumulates in the horse's chest, in addition to medical therapy, attempts are usually made to drain off the fluid. This allows the fluid to be analyzed and cultured to see what kinds of bugs are living in the horse's chest, which allows for proper antimicrobial selection. In addition, pulling the fluid out of the chest can help the horse breathe because the extra fluid compresses the lungs. Depending on how sick the horse is, there are several ways that chest drainage can be done, including needle drainage, installing a temporary drain, or in the most severe cases, even opening up the chest cavity to the outside. Some veterinarians may also choose to use the drainage site to rinse out the bugs inside the chest using large amounts of sterile fluids (the process called *lavage*).

The sooner you start to treat a horse's pleuropneumonia, the better. For example, if it is recognized that a transported horse is coming down with signs of shipping fever, it's a much better idea to get the horse to a hospital immediately, if possible, rather than continue with the transportation. You'll have a much better chance of helping the horse recover if you don't allow the disease to get firmly established.

Can pleuropneumonia be prevented?

Pleuropneumonia can be an unfortunate complication of many disease processes, all of which cause stress to the horse. In cases of severe respiratory disease or laminitis, or post-surgery, it's important to monitor the horse carefully so as to make sure that he doesn't develop a serious secondary problem.

Of course, the best way to prevent shipping fever is not to ship the horse. That's not a practical option if you're planning on going to the Olympics this year, so unfortunately, given such motivations, all you can do is try to make the best of a potentially bad situation. People do many different things in an effort to prevent shipping fever—only a few of them appear to be very important.

History can be an excellent guide. There are some rather spectacular statistics available on shipping fever from the first World War. During WWI, hundreds of horses were being lost to pleuropneumonia *each day* in the United Kingdom and the United States. Thus, the following control measures were introduced:

- Handlers were to know their charges well.
- Temperatures were routinely monitored.
- Horses did not travel if they were ill or had a fever.
- Horses were not worked for three weeks after a trip that required more than twenty-four hours to complete.
- Unnecessary stops along a journey were minimized.
- Horses were to be the last ones on transport vessels and the first ones off.

Over a twelve-month period, in an era without antibiotics, illness and mortality due to pleuropneumonia in transported horses was reduced by a staggering 80 percent on both continents. The guidelines would appear to be as appropriate today as they were then. Other things may be done—with little data to support them.

Prophylactic Antibiotics
Giving antibiotics to a horse that's going to be traveling in an effort to kill bacteria before they cause problems is not effective. Investigators in Australia gave *penicillin* prior to, and during, periods of heads-up restraint in horses and found that the only thing that giving the antibiotic did was decrease the proportion of organisms that were sensitive to penicillin. It didn't change the *total* number of organisms at all. Because there are so many different organisms found in the horse's pharynx, it would be impossible to give a single antibiotic and kill them all. In fact, if you give antibiotics to a horse prior to shipping, all that you really do is favor one kind of bug over another. So, you can most likely forget about "prophylactic" antibiotics when you're shipping your horse.

Oiling
People often worry about their horses developing colic when they are shipped. Accordingly, some people give their horses light mineral oil via a nasogastric tube prior to shipment. There's certainly no evidence that this approach helps prevent shipping-related problems, however, if you choose to have it done, you can certainly guarantee an oily mess in the transport vehicle.

Hydrating

Sometimes people try to make sure that their transported horses are well hydrated. So, they'll give these horses a bucket of water by nasogastric tube, or even intravenous fluids, before they put them onto a trailer. This probably isn't a very effective means of preventing dehydration because the horse's system rapidly gets rid of excess fluid. Of course, it's critical for a horse to have access to water during trips of any length, but giving the horse fluids before you go won't decrease the need for water along the way, nor will it prevent shipping fever.

Immune System Stimulants

A number of products are sold that purport to "stimulate" the horse's immune system. Such stimulation is, of course, considered to be good—that is, it's hoped that if the horse's immune system is "revved up," the horse will be better able to fight off disease. Unfortunately, there's nothing to suggest that these products will prevent pleuropneumonia.

What is the prognosis for horses with pleuropneumonia?

The prognosis for any horse that develops shipping fever is a bit dicey. Unless an affected horse is treated quickly and aggressively, nearly half of those diagnosed will die or will eventually be put to sleep, according to some surveys. Of those reported to survive, fewer than half can return to their previous level of work; instead, most become breeding animals or are used for such things as pleasure and trail riding. A few horses stay sick—others develop complications, such as laminitis. So, the old adage about a pound of prevention being worth a pound of cure is particularly apt with this disease.

Unfortunately, there is no way to be 100 percent sure that an individual horse will not get pleuropneumonia. While modern veterinary medicine and surgery have significantly reduced the death rate from pleuropneumonia, it is highly probable that a horse that develops the disease will not return to his prior activity level. This underscores the importance of developing the most effective strategies for its prevention. There certainly are not any magic tricks—pleuropneumonia can be a complication of many different kinds of respiratory disease. However, when healthy a horse is going to be introduced to the stress of transport, such things as briefly stopping along the way, prophylactic antibiotics, and immune system stimulants are simply no substitute for good, sensible husbandry measures and prompt recognition of any problems that occur.

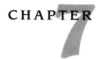

Streptococcus equi Infection ("Strangles")

Perhaps no other disease of the horse's respiratory tract invokes fear and concern like infection caused by a bacterium called *Streptococcus equi*. It must be the common name—"strangles"—that certainly invokes images of the horse succumbing to a slow and agonizing death, gasping for air. Fortunately, in almost every case, it's not that bad, especially if well managed. There are a lot of misconceptions and misunderstandings about the disease. One bacterium has created many unanswerable questions and controversies. This chapter will attempt to clarify some of them.

Which horses get strangles?

Strangles is a disease with no preference for breed, sex, or age. It is a disease of horses in herds that are easily able to come in contact with each other. Young horses seem to be particularly susceptible to outbreaks, mostly because they have had little or no chance to develop any immunity to the disease. Herded horses are the ones that can engage in normal horse social behavior, involving nuzzling and head-to-head encounters, and can thus easily transmit the disease through direct contact. However, strangles can also be transmitted indirectly, via contaminated housing, water, feed, buckets, twitches, tack, or even the clothing and equipment of handlers or veterinarians.

What causes strangles?

Strangles is caused by a bacterium from the genus *Streptococcus*, which is the same group of bacteria that causes strep throat in people. The primary source of the bacterium appears to be carrier horses. (Contrary to what some people believe, the bacterium does not live for long when it is outside of the horse.)

What are the signs of strangles?

Strangles normally causes the horse to get quite obviously sick. A horse with the disease usually stops eating, runs a fever, and develops an abundant white discharge from his nostrils. Within a few days, swelling of the *lymph nodes* under the jaw may become apparent. Initially quite firm, hot, and painful to the touch, this swelling eventually softens and forms an abscess. Once the abscess bursts (or is lanced by your veterinarian), the horse usually recovers quite rapidly, with the wound under the jaw usually requiring a couple of weeks to completely heal. Unfortunately, not all cases of strangles are simple.

What's happening in the horse?

When a horse is introduced to strangles, there's a period of three to fourteen days where the bacteria incubates inside the horse. The bacteria set up shop on the mucous membranes in the horse's nasal passages and pharynx. Initially, a horse typically develops a fever, becomes depressed, and goes off his feed. He often develops an abundant, thick discharge from his nostrils, and some horses may develop a cough or discharge from their eyes.

Once the bacteria become established, they move to local lymph nodes of the head and neck fairly quickly. The lymph node is the field where the battle between the invading bacteria and the horse's immune system takes place. As the battle rages, the lymph nodes located under the jaw and behind the ears typically become hard, swollen, and painful to the touch. Normally, these lymph nodes will abscess, drain, and heal, although other lymph nodes in the horse's body may become involved in the disease process. And, other complications may occur.

How is strangles diagnosed?

Most cases of strangles can be relatively easily diagnosed by the combination of the clinical signs of fever, nasal discharge, and swelling under the jaw. Unfortunately, not every horse presents the disease in this obvious way. For example, as outbreaks progress,

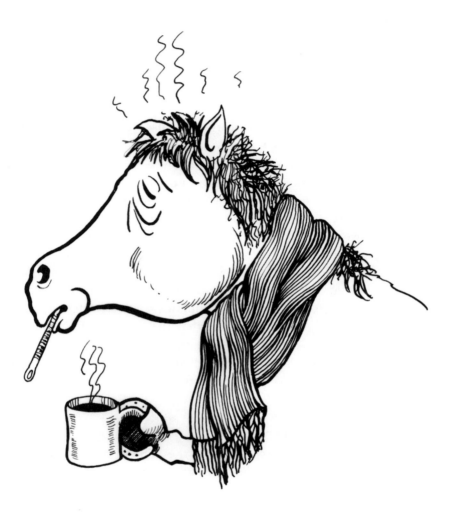

individuals may not develop the draining abscesses that characterize the disease.

A diagnosis of strangles is confirmed by isolating and growing the *S. equi* bacteria. Samples may be obtained from fluid aspirated from lymph nodes, direct culture of infected material, or swabs of the air passages. This is usually done by your veterinarian. Still, the general rule is, if it looks like strangles, it probably is strangles.

How is strangles spread?

S. equi spreads in one of two ways. The first is by direct contact, from horse to horse, either from one infected horse to another, or from a carrier horse—one that does not show signs of sickness—to a healthy horse. Unfortunately, there's no way to tell if any particular horse will become a carrier, or if he becomes a carrier, for how long he will carry the bacterium. British investigators have found horses able to carry the bacterium for over *three years*.

Strangles can also be spread by direct contact with material that has been contaminated by the strangles bacteria. When disease outbreaks occur, the environment can be a significant source of infection, as an infected horse contaminates feeders, waterers, fence posts, and the like. It's been shown that the strangles bacteria can live in soil for about three days, on a fence post for about a week, and in water for about a month. So, it's very important to make sure that such things as shared water buckets don't turn into outposts for the spread of the disease

How is strangles treated?

The "best" treatment for strangles is the subject of some controversy. It also depends on the horse's particular situation. Treatment considerations for an individual horse in a box stall may be somewhat different than handling an outbreak in a herd of yearlings. Still, most horses with strangles tend to get better on their own, and all they may need is some good nursing care. Keeping the horse in a warm, dry environment and giving him easily swallowed food can help make things easier on a sore throat. You can follow some basic principles for disease treatment and tailor the situation to your individual circumstances.

Bacteria cause strangles, and bacteria are generally susceptible to treatment with most commonly used antibiotics and antibacterials, although pencillin is considered by most veterinarians to be the antibiotic of choice. Still, the value of antibiotics in the treatment of strangles is the source of a good deal of controversy. If given early enough, before lymph node abscesses have started to form, it may be possible to keep a horse from developing that messy problem. Once the abscess has started to form, however, giving antimicrobial therapy simply delays resolution of the disease because the antibiotics can't remove pus that's already formed or easily access the bacteria within the abscesses.

In addition to antibiotic therapy, some veterinarians may choose to keep a horse's fever down using non-steroidal anti-inflammatory drugs. NSAIDs can help reduce fever, pain, and inflammation and may help the horse be more comfortable. Of course, more severe cases may require more attention; for example, the rare case may need surgical help to keep breathing by cutting a hole in the windpipe (a procedure called a *tracheostomy*).

Understandably, people get really concerned about the abscesses developing under their horses' jaws. They seem to want the abscesses to open as soon as possible, so poultices, hot towels, or smelly ointments may be applied. Whether these treatments have any real value is questionable.

What's the likely prognosis for a horse with strangles?

Most horses recover from strangles uneventfully. Their abscesses break, the skin wounds heal, and they develop some immunity to further infection, for at least the next year (they *do not* develop a life-long immunity). It's a messy disease, but usually, once it's over, it's over.

However, in some cases, horses will continue to shed the *S. equi* bacteria for a month or more after clinical signs have disappeared. These horses don't look any different from normal horses, but they can act as a source of infection for any new horse that they come in contact with. In most cases, these carrier horses harbor the strangles bacteria in their guttural pouches. Due to the fact that is not easy to get sufficient concentrations of antibiotics into the guttural pouch, direct treatment is a must if the carrier state is to be eliminated.

COMPLICATIONS OF STRANGLES

Metastatic Abscesses ("Bastard Strangles")

In some horses, the strangles bacterium does not limit itself to the lymph nodes of the head. Instead, it travels from lymph node to lymph node, abscessing its way around the horse's body. As long as the abscess is near the skin surface, repeated abscesses are mostly just messy, but when an abscess occurs deep in the body, it can be real trouble for the horse (such internal abscesses are commonly called "bastard strangles"). A horse so affected requires aggressive and long-term antibiotic or antibacterial therapy.

There's been a long-held myth that administering antibiotics to a horse with strangles will make him more likely to develop bastard strangles. There simply isn't any scientific support for such a concept. And, as noted, if a horse does develop an internal abscess, the treatment is antibiotics.

Purpura Hemorrhagica

Purpura is an acute complication of strangles that's caused by the horse's immune system going wild. It's usually seen in the older horse. The disease is characterized by inflamed blood vessels and dramatic swelling of the horse's body, particularly his head and legs. Inflamed blood vessels can be anywhere in the horse, so many organs, including the heart, muscles, and intestines can become affected. The swelling can be bad enough to cause circulatory collapse and death.

The treatment of purpura is aimed at calming the horse's immune system and controlling the blood vessel inflammation and swelling. Typically, corticosteroid drugs are used to do this, and non-steroidal anti-inflammatory drugs may be used to help control the fever, as well. Antibiotic therapy is also commonly used, however, some veterinarians feel that antibiotics should be avoided in purpura horses because the immune system may be further stimulated as bacteria are killed and released into the horse's system. Supportive care to get rid of the fluid, such as exercise, leg bandages, and water therapy, may also be useful.

Strep Mysositis

The term *myositis* refers to inflammation of the muscles, in particular, the skeletal muscles that make the horse's body move. A horse affected with myositis is typically quite sore to the touch and may be lame. Following *S. equi* infections, two different syndromes are recognized.

The first type of strep myositis is associated with purpura hemorrhagica. The inflammation of the surface blood vessels that characterizes purpura extends to the muscles themselves. These cases can be confused with horses that "tie up" after intense exercise. The second strep myositis most often occurs in young to young adult Quarter Horses. In these horses, exposure to the *S. equi* bacteria can cause skeletal muscle damage and rapid muscle wasting, even when there haven't been obvious signs of infection. Both conditions may require some time for full recovery and may benefit from good supportive care by you and your veterinarian.

Can strangles be prevented?

Typically, disease prevention involves two different strategies. One is management—the other is vaccination. Management is demonstrably useful in preventing strangles, but the available vaccines have provoked controversies.

Management techniques, such as isolation of a new horse for a period of two to four weeks prior to introducing him into an established herd, may be useful in preventing the introduction of respiratory disease into a population. In addition, identification and treatment of carrier horses is especially helpful at controlling outbreaks of strangles. Unfortunately, identifying carriers isn't all that simple. Weekly swabs of nasal and pharyngeal areas for bacterial culture and DNA testing can help—rinsing both guttural pouches four to six weeks after an active infection has ended appears to be an even more sensitive method of detection. So, stable owners can consider trying to identify carrier horses when they first enter the stable, particularly if they have been previously ill. Whether this approach is economical is a decision that each individual must make.

It would be great if you could prevent a horse from becoming a carrier in the first place. Unfortunately, that's not all that easy, either.

Some veterinarians routinely put a horse on antibiotics after his strangles abscesses have opened, both to try to prevent the spread of the bacteria through the system and to prevent carriers; however, there's little evidence that this approach is successful, perhaps in part because the bacteria can hide in the guttural pouches, away from the blood circulation and the antibiotics that travel in it. A combination of guttural pouch lavage and antibiotics might help eliminate carriers, but again, the cost of treating every horse may not be worth the benefit.

Environmental management is critical for successful control of strangles. In most cases, all horses coming into and out of a facility with an outbreak should be held, pending control of the disease. Horses that are infected should be kept away from other horses. In the face of a strangles outbreak, barn surfaces should be kept clean, tack and equipment shouldn't be shared, and water buckets and troughs should be scrubbed regularly. People shouldn't handle infected horses and then come into contact with healthy ones—that just increases the potential spread of the disease.

There are two types of vaccines available for the prevention of strangles in the United States—the *intramuscular (IM)* and the *intranasal (IN)* vaccine; however, the fact is that very few nations currently use vaccination as a means of preventing the disease. Even in the U.S., where the vaccines are often used, strangles remains a significant problem.

Unfortunately, none of the vaccines used for the prevention of strangles—neither those administered intramuscularly, nor those given intranasally—are supported by good data from large trials showing that they actually prevent the disease. The immunity provoked by the vaccines is both poor and short-lived. Because of complications such as fever, swelling, pain at the site of injection (in the case of IM), and the possibility of introducing vaccine-related disease (if the vaccine is administered IN), some veterinarians feel that the vaccines are just as bad as the disease.

The intranasal vaccine, in particular, should be handled and administered with careful consideration. The vaccine is a live bacterium, and cases of strangles—in addition to milder complications, such as fever or nasal discharge—that have been caused by the vaccine strain of the bacteria have been identified. Intramuscular abscesses have been identified in horses that have received other vaccinations at the same time that the strangles vaccine was administered—this appears to have been caused by spreading the administered vaccine onto the skin along with introducing the bacteria into the muscle by a subsequent vaccination. If you do choose to use this type of vaccine, make sure that it is given alone, or in the case of multiple shots, as the last one.

Considerable controversy surrounds whether vaccines should be administered to horses in the face of an outbreak of strangles. The reasons to do so are perhaps obvious—if an immune response can be mounted early enough, some horses may be able to fight off the disease without developing clinical signs. However, there are numerous reasons to consider avoiding vaccination in the face of disease. In the first place, a vaccine-related immune response is unlikely to occur fast enough to help fight off an infection that is running through a herd. Secondly, attempting to provoke an aggressive immune response to a disease such as strangles may lead to the development of complications, such as purpura. More of something *is not* necessarily better.

Inflammatory Disease of the Lower Airway ("Heaves")

"**H**eaves" (also referred to as *chronic obstructive pulmonary disease*, "broken wind," *bronchiolitis*, or *recurrent airway obstruction*, among other monikers) is a common disease of the horse's lower airway. Almost undoubtedly, it's the most common respiratory problem affecting mature, stabled horses. It's an environmental disease that causes a reversible narrowing of the small air passages, with alternating periods of remission and disease.

Which horses get heaves?

Heaves is most commonly seen when the horse is stabled inside where the circulation of air may not be ideal. It's also seen in locations where it can be difficult to find adequately dry hay. If hay isn't completely dried, it can become moldy and dusty—mold and dust are the sort of things that trigger the difficult breathing episodes that characterize the disease. Of course, often, the same climatic conditions that require the horse to be stabled inside preclude thorough drying of hay, so there's probably some overlap. It's a fact that heaves is also sometimes seen in horses that are kept at pasture year-round, but most often, it's a disease of older, mature horses that are kept indoors for much of the time. There also seem to be some breed-related and hereditary aspects of the disease—no preference for gender has been seen—but the details of such aspects have not yet been worked out.

What causes heaves?

It's generally felt that several things—perhaps several things working together at the same time, and all affecting the horse's air passages—set off an allergic-type reaction that leads to the characteristic clinical signs of heaves. Horses have apparently been getting heaves since horse medicine was first described—Aristotle may have even recognized the condition. Heaves was linked to poor-quality hay fairly early on. Originally, it was thought that bad hay packed up in the intestines and put pressure on the horse's diaphragm, causing respiratory difficulties (that's *not* what happens). However, it wasn't long before mold and dust were recognized to be triggering factors for the disease. Other factors were also noted, for example, an association between the heavey horse and stables near chickens has been made. In addition, some people think that viral infection may cause a horse to develop heaves (the same sort of thing has been seen in human asthma).

What are the signs of heaves?

A horse affected with inflammation of his lower airway can show signs varying from an inability to exercise normally and a mild cough early in the disease, to a severe, full-blown respiratory crisis, where the horse is literally gasping for air in a long-term case. In that regard, the clinical appearance can be much like that of asthma or emphysema in people, although these are actually quite different from the disease that occurs in horses. Nevertheless, due to such similarities, some people may erroneously refer to a horse with heaves as having "equine asthma."

A horse affected with heaves shows clinical signs because the lower air passages narrow or constrict. Narrow air passages make it hard for air to move in and out of the lungs of the affected horse. The smaller the air passages (the more constriction occurs as a result of the condition) the harder it is for the horse to get air through them. Think of trying to move water through a pipe. The bigger the pipe, the easier it is for the water to flow through it, and vice versa.

It's this difficulty in moving air that gives the disease its common name. A severely affected horse stands with his chest "heaving," trying to get some precious air in and out. Other common signs of heaves include coughing and/or a whitish discharge coming from the nostrils. The nostrils of the affected horse may flare open with the effort of each breath. Over time, a "heave line" can develop along the horse's belly, caused by all of the work that the horse has to do with his abdominal muscles to assist the chest with the effort of

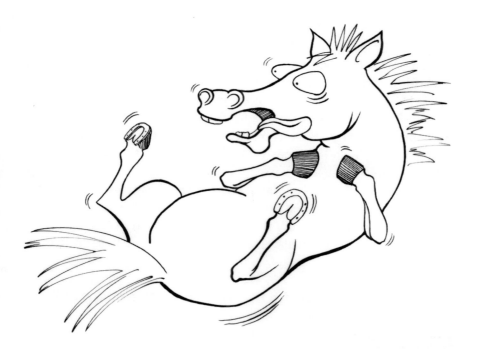

breathing. In a severe case, the horse may lose weight—even become emaciated—due to the constant effort and work required to breathe.

All along the airways in a heavy horse, your veterinarian may hear signs of problems (they are usually best heard with a stethoscope). The windpipe (or trachea) may be full of secretions, which can cause a noisy, turbulent sound. Inside the horse's chest, all sorts of weird sounds occur as a result of the problem, from wheezes to crackles and high-pitched whistles, to areas of eerie silence where the air isn't flowing well at all. In early cases, listening to the chest may not provide much of a symphony, so your veterinarian might put a bag over the horse's nose for a minute or so, prior to examining him. As was discussed in chapter 2, rebreathing the expired carbon dioxide that collects in the bag makes the horse breathe harder when the bag is removed (you can't ask a horse to take a deep breath), and breathing harder makes the airway sounds more distinct. However, this isn't necessary in more severe cases.

The signs of disease in a heavy horse are often fairly easy to recognize. Usually, if not treated appropriately, the signs may worsen over time. The signs may also change with the seasons; for example, they may be worse in winter, when the horse is kept indoors in a poorly ventilated barn. The heavy breathing may become more exaggerated when an afflicted horse is fed poor-quality hay or kept in dusty conditions. These signs are often reversible when the horse is in a well-ventilated situations, such as out in good pasture.

What's happening in the horse's air passages?

When a horse with heaves is exposed to the things that trigger the disease, three things happen. First, the airways become inflamed. Second, the bronchi and brochioles, the air passages that wind through the lungs, constrict. Third, mucus is produced.

Inflammation

Inflammation is a normal, local, protective response of the horse's body to irritation, injury, or infection, but in the lungs, it leads to a loss of normal lung function. The inflammatory process causes large numbers of white blood cells to enter the air passages, cells that release a variety of chemicals in an effort to take care of the agents that set off the disease process. The presence or absence of such cells can be helpful diagnostically, as well.

Bronchoconstriction

The air passages through the lungs are surrounded with a special type of muscle called *smooth muscle*. The presence of muscle allows the air passages to be *dynamic*—they can open or close depending on circumstances. For example, air passages dilate when a horse is exercising and needs as much oxygen as he can get; this allows for more air to be able to pass into the lungs. The reason that the air passages constrict in a horse with heaves is not fully known, but it is known that some of the chemicals released in the process of inflammation can cause constriction.

Mucus Production and Accumulation

Another problem that occurs with heaves is the accumulation of mucus in the air passages. In a long-term, severe case of heaves, sticky mucous plugs can sit in the airway and essentially block the passage of air. They can even make it impossible for drugs to get in and help fight the disease.

The combination of inflammation, constricted bronchi, and mucus buildup in the air passages blocks the flow of air into the lungs and leads to a lack of oxygen in the horse's blood. A horse that has heaves can't ventilate his lungs normally—this means that a greater respiratory effort than normal is required to get oxygen into the horse's body. In long-standing cases, heaves can even cause permanent changes in the lungs, such as scarring or an increase in the size of the cells in the smooth muscle around the air passages. Once changes like these have occurred, it's essentially impossible to do anything about them, and a horse in this situation can be very difficult to treat.

How is heaves diagnosed?

You can usually get some idea that a horse has heaves based on clinical signs. After all, it's usually pretty hard to overlook a horse that's gasping for air. Still, there are other diseases that make a horse gasp for air so clinical signs may not be all that you need to come up with a firm diagnosis. It's pretty important to make sure that a correct diagnosis is made before treatment is given.

That said, an older horse with a history that includes things like being confined in a poorly ventilated, indoor stable and being given bad hay, accompanied by a clinical exam that finds wheezing and crackling lungs, often allows for a pretty secure diagnosis of heaves. Young horses typically don't get heaves—they're better candidates for temporary inflammation of the lower airway or an infectious disease, such as pneumonia. A horse with heaves usually doesn't have the fever that tends to accompany infection. Blood tests are often unremarkable, but they're useful because a normal blood test helps rule out deep-seated infection as a cause of breathing problems.

It may be necessary for more detailed diagnostic efforts to determine if a more subtly affected horse has heaves. For example, techniques to obtain cell samples from the lungs, such as bronchoalveolar lavage or transtracheal aspiration biopsy (a "tracheal wash") may be extremely helpful in coming up with a diagnosis. Giving a test dose of a drug to dilate the bronchi, such as injecting *atropine* intravenously, can help confirm the presence of constricted bronchi. Radiographs (X rays) are generally less helpful in highlighting the fibrous tissue that can build up in the horse's lungs, but may be recommended. Endoscopy, where the veterinarian looks down the horse's air passages with a fiberoptic scope, usually only shows accumulations of mucus, though it's also possible to obtain diagnostic specimens through the endoscope. Arterial blood gas examinations may show a decreased amount of oxygen in the horse's blood as a result of poor airway function. These exams are not particularly difficult for trained veterinarians to perform and don't really pose any undue risk to the horse's health. The information obtained from them may be invaluable.

On the other hand, lung biopsies, while certainly a fairly reliable method of determining problems in the lung, also carry the risk of severe bleeding and are generally not recommended for evaluating a heavey horse. Allergen testing, whether by means of a skin prick test or blood serum analysis, is also of questionable value.

How is heaves treated?

The bedrock of successful heaves treatment has been environmental management, in particular, dust control and good ventilation. In fact, studies have shown that the single most effective treatment for heaves is to keep the infected horse's setting as dust-free and well aired as possible. There's no substitute for good management. Unfortunately, good management may not be easy, and some people are much more willing and able to give medical treatment than they are to correct the underlying problems in a horse's surroundings.

Several sources of dust may need to be addressed. First of all, the horse's hay must be of good quality. The horse spends a good bit of his day eating and breathing-in hay dust. His muzzle is right down in and on the hay. All sorts of mold and fungi, as well as dust, can be present in poor-quality hay. The simplest solution to this problem is for the horse to get his nutrients from a pasture, but of course, this isn't always possible, particularly if it's winter and the ground is covered with snow. So, you may need to look for other solutions.

One good way to keep dust down is to soak hay in water. "Soaking" means to put a flake of hay underwater for several minutes, until it is thoroughly wet; merely hosing a hay flake, or sprinkling some water on top of it, is unlikely to be of much use. Unfortunately, soaking hay is labor intensive (people may get tired of doing it) and may decrease the nutritional content of the hay. There's also the green water to dispose of—clearly, hay-soaking is not the answer for everyone. There are alternatives.

Kiln-dried hay may be available in your area and is a good substitute for hay that's been properly dried in the field. Hay pellets—even complete pelleted diets—can usually be purchased for a reasonable cost, and they typically are not dusty and don't contain mold or spores. Silage, which is prepared by storing and fermenting green forage plants, can also be a good feed, but you have to be very careful with it. Cow silage is prone to developing *botulinum toxin,* to which the horse is extremely sensitive, so it may not be appropriate. Good quality, commercial silage is probably preferable to the made-on-the-farm stuff.

The next important source of dust and mold in the horse's environment is bedding. Bedding shouldn't be too wet because it will be hard to clean and promotes mold, but it shouldn't be too dusty, either. Wood shavings are probably better than straw because straw tends to have more mold than shavings. Other bedding alternatives are available, such as rice hulls, paper, cardboard, and peat moss.

However, they also may have drawbacks, such as difficulty in disposal and/or a tendency of the horse to eat his bedding and develop intestinal problems (colic, for example).

Good ventilation is extremely important in barns but can never take the place of good stall management. No matter how good the ventilation system is, it still can't remove the dust and mold the horse comes into contact with through his feed. Still, good ventilation is certainly something to strive for, particularly because other horse owners may not be as fastidious about managing their stalls as you are about yours. Good airflow can help keep *some* of the dust down.

To sum things up, here are ten things that you can do to make your horse's environment more healthy for his airway.

1. Try to house your horse in a stall that allows him to hang his head outside.
2. Consider placing a fan in the stall (safely secured and out of the horse's reach) to move air.
3. Feed hay near or on the ground, rather that in a high hayrack or net. In hayracks, particles easily get into your horse's eyes and nostrils.
4. Consider soaking hay in water before feeding, or use low-dust alternatives, such as hay cubes.
5. Sprinkle barn aisles and stalls with water after you sweep, rake, or clean.
6. Store hay and bedding away from your horse.
7. Dispose of hay, feed, or bedding that shows signs of mold.
8. Use a moisture-and odor-absorbing product, such as lime, on the floor of stalls.
9. Keep old bedding and manure piles away from your horse and remove them from your property regularly.
10. Let your horse live outside as much as possible.

MEDICATIONS FOR HEAVES

Corticosteroids

The most common, and the most effective, medications used in the treatment of heaves are corticosteroid drugs. These drugs are the only ones that directly counteract inflammation in the horse's lower air passages that occur as a result of the disease.

Most commonly, corticosteroids such as *dexamethasone* and *triamcinolone* have been given by injection or orally to control heaves. *Prednisone*, a corticosteroid that is commonly used for the treatment of a number of conditions of small animals (and humans) appears not to be well utilized by horses and probably isn't the best choice of drug; its cousin, *prednisolone*, would appear to be a better choice.

Corticosteroids are notorious in some species (including people) for a variety of side effects. In horses, many of those effects, such as weight gain, appear to be largely absent. However, there seems to be a general concern about the possible connection between use of these drugs—particularly the more potent and long-lasting ones most commonly used for heaves treatment—and the development of laminitis (inflammation of the connections that bind the horse's foot to his hoof). While such an association has been suggested, no one has ever been able to demonstrate it in experimental trials. Nevertheless, when using oral or injectable corticosteroids, it's probably a good idea to control the disease using the lowest dose as infrequently as possible. Most therapeutic schemes for use of the drugs involve more frequent administration initially, with decreasing doses as therapy is maintained in the long-term.

Perhaps the safest and most effective way of administering corticosteroids is via aerosol preparations. Inhalers are undoubtedly the most common method of application in humans that require corticosteroids for the control of their respiratory problems. Inhalers provide several advantages for corticosteroid administration. First of all, the medication is administered directly into the air passages. Second, the doses used in treatment are small, relative to the larger doses required when corticosteroids are given orally or by injection. Third, when given by the aerosol route, much less of the drug is absorbed by the horse, thus greatly decreasing any risk of side effects. Some aerosol medications, however, may cause a horse to test positive if he is screened for drugs.

Unfortunately, it's a bit more involved to get a horse to take inhaled medication than it is to get a human to do so. The aerosol mask made specifically for a horse[1] (see page 26) slips over the horse's

---

1 Equine Aeromask™; Trudell Medical International, London, Ontario, Canada

muzzle and allows the drug to be administered via a chamber from which the horse breathes. There's also a device that can be placed over one of the horse's nostrils that does the same sort of thing.[2] While these devices are somewhat expensive, they're probably worth purchasing to control chronic cases, or if you have several horses to treat. Oral or injectable forms of corticosteroids can certainly be effective, and when choosing a method of treatment, the determining factor for some people is the cost of the necessary medication.

Bronchodilators

When treating heaves, some people may employ drugs that try to open the horse's constricted air passages. Relieving the spasm of the bronchi is a laudable goal, as it should improve the passage of air into the horse's lungs. That's almost certainly a good thing, particularly if the disease is severe or the horse is in respiratory crisis. Some people have also given bronchodilators prior to giving corticosteroids in hopes that by dilating the bronchi, more of the corticosteroid drug will get into the lungs.

That said, it's probably not a good idea to use bronchodilators as the sole form of therapy for a heavey horse. In the first place, bronchoconstriction is largely a result of inflammation, and treating the bronchoconstriction without treating the inflammation is pretty futile. Secondly, using such drugs without making changes in the horse's environment probably isn't a great idea—you sure don't want to relax the horse's airways only to increase the amount of material getting into them.

Atropine is probably the most effective drug known to relax constricted air passages. Unfortunately, it's a drug that can also have some fairly severe complications on the gastrointestinal effects, shutting down normal intestinal movement and causing colic. Because of this, atropine is mostly used in test doses to see if a horse's airway responds. Drugs such as *ipratropium bromide* can be given via the aerosol route, or *clenbuterol* can be administered orally. Other drugs, such as *theophylline* or *albuterol*, may be advocated for oral use in a heavey horse, but their absorption may be poor or their margin of safety may be narrow. Accordingly, they probably aren't the best choices.

2 Equine Haler, Jorgensen Laboratories, Loveland, CO, USA.

Other Medications

It would make sense to try to loosen up the mucus in the air passages of a horse with heaves; however, there isn't really any good evidence to suggest that there's a practical way to do this. *Guaifenesin*, a medication commonly used in human over-the-counter cough preparations to promote the expulsion of mucus, hasn't been shown to have much effectiveness in people, much less horses. Drugs such as *acetylcysteine*, or even saline, administered via aerosol in an effort to loosen respiratory secretions, haven't been shown to work in horses. People have tried to "hyperhydrate" heavey horses—that is, give them large volumes of intravenous fluids—but this was shown to be an ineffective form of treatment, as well. Antihistamines have been often used for the treatment of heaves, although there is essentially no evidence that they are effective. Immunostimulants, as well as non-steroidal anti-inflammatory drugs, such as phenylbutazone, appear to have little use in heaves treatment. Antibiotics are only indicated when a concurrent infection exists. Finally, cough suppressants should probably not be used in a horse with heaves because coughing is a necessary means by which the horse clears the mucous secretions from his lungs.

"Alternative" Approaches

As with any disease without an immediate cure, or when side effects of drugs are feared, alternatives to conventional, effective treatments may exist. While unlikely to be of much harm, there's essentially no evidence that they are effective. For example, acupuncture has been shown to be ineffective for the management of human asthma, and manual therapies, such as chiropractic, have failed to demonstrate that they have any relevant effects on lung function in human asthma, as well.

The use of plants is perhaps the oldest known form of human therapy, and plant-based remedies are available for heaves treatment. Perceptions that pharmaceutical medications are expensive, overprescribed, and dangerous may drive people to herbal therapies that may be perceived as "natural" and therefore safe, but whether they are effective is another question. In people, herbal remedies have not been shown to be effective treatments for asthmatics. The effects of an oral preparation containing an extract of thyme and primula on the lung function of five horses suffering heaves found that the product did not improve their clinical signs, nor did it increase the amount of oxygen in the horses' arteries.

One study suggested that a supplement consisting of a mixture of natural antioxidants, including vitamins E and C, and selenium from a variety of sources, was effective at modulating airway inflammation in heavey horses, although markers of lung function and the results of bronchoalveolar lavage testing were not significantly affected. That said, if the most effective and most "natural" treatment for heaves—environmental management—is applied, just about any other adjunctive therapy will most likely appear to work.

What is the likely prognosis for horses with heaves?

Some people have used test doses of atropine to try to help determine the prognosis for a heavy horse—if the horse fails to respond to atropine administration, the prognosis may be poor. However, in reality, there are few reports of long-term outcomes and management of heavey horses. Good environmental management plays a critical role in a successful outcome, however, studies have shown that people routinely fail to employ or maintain the recommendations for changing the conditions that cause the problem in the first place. That's really too bad, because with some effort on the part of their owners, most horses with heaves can be helped.

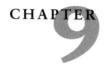

Exercise-Induced Pulmonary Hemorrhage ("Bleeding")

The bleeding from the horse's lungs that can occur during exercise (*exercise-induced pulmonary hemorrhage* or *EIPH*) is one of the major causes of decreased athletic performance in horses of various disciplines. In the United States, many horses are treated prior to performing with substances designed to prevent lung bleeding, including (somewhat controversially) many racehorses. EIPH is a concern for the horse's health, as well as an economic concern for the horse owner.

Which horses get EIPH?

The horses most commonly observed to bleed from their lungs are racehorses, including Thoroughbreds, Standardbreds, and Quarter Horses. However, just about any horse that exercises intensely can bleed, and the condition has been seen in field hunters, event horses, jumpers, barrel racers, cutters, and polo horses—even draft horses have been affected. Bleeding seems to be more a function of the intensity of exercise than the duration; it's not something that's commonly seen among endurance horses, for example. Most studies have failed to show that there's any sort of a sex predilection for EIPH, and there doesn't seem to be a genetic component, either. However, bleeding does seem to be more of a problem in older horses than in younger ones.

What causes EIPH?

The understanding of EIPH has come along slowly. It was once felt that the bleeding occurred in the head, and it wasn't until the early 1970s that it was first noted that the blood actually came from the horse's lungs. A number of theories have been proposed in an effort to understand why EIPH occurs.

Initially, people proposed that a horse bled from areas of the lung that were weakened by previous disease. So, for example, they felt that a horse that had a previous episode of pneumonia was more likely to become a bleeder because scar tissue in the horse's lungs would be more likely to tear and bleed than normal tissue. However, this has not been shown to be the case. Nor have any of the other theories as to the cause of EIPH—upper airway obstruction, changes in blood thickness with exercise, lower airway disease, or even mechanical pressure waves from the hooves striking the ground (swimming horses have been reported to bleed)—been shown to be true.

The most current theory is that lung blood vessels rupture because of stress in an exercising horse. During exercise, the lung blood vessels undergo extreme pressure changes. These changes, in addition to the heavy, deep breathing required for intense exercise, may simply rupture the small blood vessels of the lungs. As such, EIPH may be an inevitable consequence of intense exercise in some horses.

What are the signs of EIPH?

The most obvious clinical sign of a "bleeder" is blood in the nostrils after exercise. However, looking for blood in the nostrils is not necessarily the best way to diagnose the condition, and relatively few horses that bleed from their lungs get a bloody nose. Tests done with flexible fiberoptic endoscopes, which allow veterinarians to look down into the horse's air passages, disturbingly report that as many as 75 to 100 percent of horses may bleed from their lungs after intense exercise.

One episode of EIPH may not be a problem for a horse, but repeated episodes can be. If a horse bleeds repeatedly from his lungs, long-term lung damage can result. The horse so affected may not be able to exercise to his full capabilities, as fibrous scar tissue replaces normal lung tissue. In addition, damaged lung may become prone to further episodes of bleeding, leading to a vicious cycle. Damaged lung may also be an entry point for disease-causing organisms, and pneumonia, following episodes of bleeding, has been reported. Finally, in the most severe cases, a horse can actually bleed to death.

What happens in the horse's air passages?

Although it's perhaps obvious, a horse that bleeds from his lungs due to ruptured blood vessels has bloody lungs. The extent to which the discoloration and damage occurs depends on the extent of the bleeding—for unknown reasons, the parts of the lungs closer to the horse's back seem to be more likely to bleed than other parts. Areas of lung that have bled inflate more slowly than normal lung tissue. Bleeding causes lung inflammation, as well. Fibrous scar tissue can develop in areas where repeated episodes have occurred. All of these things serve to impair the normal function of the lungs. In addition, when bleeding occurs during exercise, the blood can essentially fill up part of the lungs, making it difficult for the horse to breathe. That's one of the primary reasons a horse with EIPH may not perform well.

How is EIPH diagnosed?

Some cases of EIPH are pretty easy to diagnose—just look at the horse's nose! As previously noted, endoscopes have greatly improved the diagnostic capabilities of veterinarians and have allowed them to diagnose the majority of cases that are less obvious. Endoscopes are relatively affordable and readily available, and thus, they are the primary tools used to make a diagnosis of EIPH. Techniques for washing the air passages, such as bronchoalveolar lavage (BAL) or transtracheal aspiration biopsy ("tracheal wash"), are diagnostic because they show the presence of blood cells in the air passages, but they are more invasive and may not be necessary in most cases. On the other hand, radiographs (X rays) of the lungs are not very useful for confirming a diagnosis of the condition.

How is EIPH treated?

It's likely that there are just about as many treatments for EIPH as there are people treating the condition. There's a pretty good rule that applies to such situations: when there are dozens of different treatments, it's likely that none of them work very well. Accordingly, if your horse has EIPH, it's likely that he will be treated according to what the attending veterinarian believes to most likely be successful.

One important factor that can be managed in a horse with EIPH is the environment. Sometimes in a horse with heaves, or with another inflammatory condition of the airway, the pressure across the small blood vessels of the lungs (the capillaries) may be greater than normal because he has to work harder to breathe normally. A horse with increased pressure on these vessels may be likely to bleed, and if he does bleed, he may bleed more severely than others. Thus, a horse with allergic or inflammatory disease of the lungs may ship into a bad stall environment and then start to have problems with EIPH. Even a normal horse may develop airway problems when put in a bad environment. Removing a horse from a bad environment or treating allergic signs can improve the horse's performance and significantly decrease the occurrence of EIPH.

MEDICATIONS FOR EIPH

The most commonly used drug for the treatment of EIPH is called *furosemide*,[3] and it's been used to treat EIPH horses for more than 30 years. Racehorses in the United States and Canada may be treated with furosemide, usually anywhere from 30 minutes to four hours before racing.

Furosemide is a *diuretic*. Diuretic agents tend to increase the flow of urine. Furosemide is used for the treatment of bleeders because it's been shown to help decrease the pressures in the blood vessels that normally increase with exercise. It does appear to be somewhat effective, at least in the lab; lab studies have shown a decrease in lung bleeding in horses exercising on a treadmill when they were given the drug. However, for unknown reasons, such effects have not been as remarkable in horses examined after they've finished racing. Regardless, the use of furosemide in performance horses is somewhat controversial because the drug has been shown to improve athletic performance, but whether this is because of direct effects on EIPH, or because of other effects, such as a decrease in water weight after the horse urinates, is unknown.

As previously noted, if furosemide were all that great at preventing lung bleeding, there wouldn't be any need for other treatments. But there's a real smorgasbord out there. The more popular ones include:
- nebulization with water-saturated air.

3 Lasix™, Aventis Pharmaceuticals

- *estrogens* (thought to improve blood vessel stability).
- *cromolyn sodium* (a drug that stablizes the membranes of certain inflammatory cells, most commonly used for the treatment of allergies in people).
- *caproic acid* or *Amicar* (a drug used in humans to control bleeding caused by the inability of the blood to form stable clots. This may also be used in conjunction with furosemide.)
- innumerable herbal or nutritional supplements, all of which have failed to demonstrate efficacy.

A more recent, non-drug treatment for bleeders is the use of *nasal dilating strips*.[4] You see these on people who use them to prevent snoring, or on football players, who use them to try to get their nostrils to open up and allow more air into their lungs. Those who advocate the strips say that they work by decreasing the resistance to air flow that's caused by the horse's nostrils—by opening the nostrils, air is supposed to flow more easily when the horse breathes, making him less likely to bleed. Studies on the strips have suggested that they both help and don't help horses with EIPH (that is, the studies conflict). They're prohibited by some racing jurisdictions.

Another approach to EIPH involves the use of *nitric oxide* or similar compounds. These agents cause blood vessels to dilate—dilated blood vessels would presumably have less pressure in them than constricted ones. As with most EIPH therapies, conflicting reports exist as to the effectiveness of such agents, however, one study indicated that the blood count in the lungs was actually doubled after exercising horses breathed-in nitric oxide.

What is the likely prognosis for horses with EIPH?

EIPH is a condition that affects virtually every horse, in every discipline that requires intense exercise. As repeated episodes occur, the affected parts of the lung become inflamed. Chronic inflammation and bleeding can lead to permanent lung changes, which in turn can lead to decreased performance, or worse, infection or even death. A horse may not bleed from the same place, or to the same extent,

---

4 Flair™ nasal strips, CNS, Inc., Minneapolis, MN

with every episode of exercise. Unfortunately, the available diagnostic procedures are not extremely sensitive and don't allow veterinarians to determine how much lung damage has actually been done. Furthermore, since no treatment has been shown to be uniformly, or even consistently, effective, it isn't currently possible to prevent EIPH by any other means than decreasing the intensity of the horse's exercise. Thus, for some horses, EIPH may be a career-ender. Cure of the condition awaits future developments.

AFTERWORD

The horse's respiratory system can be difficult to understand and treat, for veterinarians and horse owners alike. Veterinary medicine has made significant advances over the years, but there is much more knowledge yet to come. Some diseases, such as many of the types of respiratory infection to which the horse is susceptible, can be treated fairly effectively. Others, such as exercise-induced pulmonary hemorrhage, have yet to find consistently effective treatments. Sometimes, surgery may be needed to correct problems with your horse's respiratory tract, and techniques such as lasers and new surgical interventions hold the promise of even greater success in the future.

Prevention is always the best option—an ounce of it is worth *at least* a pound of cure. Proper vaccination schedules, developed with the help of your veterinarian and devised with your horse's particular circumstances in mind, can play an important role in keeping your horse healthy. In addition, management of the horse's environment plays an important role in the prevention and treatment of many of the most common conditions affecting the horse—you should always keep in mind that attacking a disease condition without looking at all of the potential underlying causes is an exercise that is bound to be futile.

If you take good care of your horse, it's not likely that serious respiratory disease is going to be a problem for him. Unfortunately, disease does happen, even under the best of circumstances. Through it all, remember that medicine is a rational endeavor and the best approach to disease of the horse's respiratory tract is thoughtful and based on sound principles of therapy. Your horse deserves nothing less.

BIBLIOGRAPHY

Ainsworth, D.M. and R.P. Hackett. "Disorders of the Respiratory System."
  Equine Internal Medicine, 2nd ed., S.M. Reed, W.M. Bayly, and D.C. Sellon,
  2nd ed., St. Louis, MO: W.B. Saunders, 2004: 289–353.

Barr, B.S. "Pneumonia in Weanlings." *Vet. Clin. NA Eq. Practice*. 2003; 19(1): 35–50.

Birks, E.K., M.M. Duando, and S. McBride. "Exercise-Induced Pulmonary
  Hemorrhage." *Vet Clin NA Eq Practice*, 2003; 19(1): 87–100.

Davenport-Goodall, C.L.M. and E.J. Parente. "Disorders of the Larynx."
  Vet Clin NA Eq Practice, 2003; 19(1): 69–188.

Flaminio, M.J.B.F. "Immunomodulators in Respiratory Disease Treatment."
  Current Therapy in Equine Medicine 5, by N.E.
  Robinson, ed, St. Louis, MO: W.B. Saunders, 2003: 445–449.

Freeman, D.E. "Sinus Disease." *Vet Clin NA Eq Practice*, 2003; 19(1): 209–244.

Hardy, J. and R. Leveille. "Diseases of the Guttural Pouches."
  Vet. Clin. NA Eq. Practice, 2003; 19(1): 123–159.

Hoffman, A.M. "Inflammatory Airway Diseases: Definitions and Diagnosis in the
  Performance Horse," *Current Therapy in Equine Medicine 5*, N.E. Robinson, ed.,
  St. Louis, MO: W.B. Saunders, 2003: 412– 417.

Kraus, B.M. and E.J. Parente. "Laryngeal Hemiplegia in Non-Racehorses."
  Current Therapy in Equine Medicine 5, N.E. Robinson, ed., St. Louis, MO: W.B.
  Saunders, 2003: 383–386.

Lavoie, J.P. "Heaves (Recurrent Airway Obstruction): Practical Management of
  Acute Episodes and Prevention of Exacerbations." *Current Therapy in Equine
  Medicine 5*, N.E. Robinson, ed., St. Louis, MO: W.B. Saunders, 2003: 417–421.

Leguillette, R. "Recurrent Airway Obstruction—Heaves." *Vet. Clin. NA Eq. Practice*,
  2003; 19(1): 63–86.

Marlin, D.J. "Exercise-Induced Pulmonary Hemorrhage." *Current Therapy in Equine Medicine 5*, N.E. Robinson, ed., St. Louis, MO: W.B. Saunders, 2003: 429–433.

Mazan, M. "Use of Aerosolized Bronchodilators and Corticosteroids." *Current Therapy in Equine Medicine 5*, N.E. Robinson, ed., St. Louis, MO: W.B. Saunders, 2003: 440–445.

Parente, E.J. "Endoscopic Evaluation of the Upper Respiratory Tract." *Current Therapy in Equine Medicine 5*, N.E. Robinson, ed., St. Louis, MO: W.B. Saunders, 2003: 366–369.

Roy, M.F. and J.P. Lavoie. "Tools for the Diagnosis of Equine Respiratory Disorders." *Vet. Clin. NA Eq. Practice*, 2003; 19(1): 1–18.

Rush, B.R. "Aerosolized Drug Delivery Devices." *Current Therapy in Equine Medicine 5*, N.E. Robinson, ed., St. Louis, MO: W.B. Saunders, 2003: 436–440.

Sprayberry, K.A. and T.D. Byars. "Equine Pleuropneumonia." *Eq. Vet. Ed.* 1999; 1: 160–164.

Sullivan, E.K. and E.J. Parente. "Disorders of the Pharynx." *Vet. Clin. NA Eq. Practice*, 2003; 19(1): 159–168.

Sweeney, C.R. "Pleuropneumonia." *Current Therapy in Equine Medicine 5*, N.E. Robinson, ed., St. Louis, MO: W.B. Saunders, 2003: 421–424.

Wilkins, P.A. "Lower Respiratory Problems of the Neonate." *Vet. Clin. NA Eq. Practice*, 2003; 19(1): 19–34.

Wilkins, P.A. "Lower Airway Diseases of the Adult Horse." *Vet. Clin. NA Eq. Practice*, 2003; 19(1): 101–122.

INDEX

Page numbers in *italic* indicate illustrations.

Acetylcysteine, 79
Acupuncture, 32, 79
Administering drugs, 23–27, *26*
Adult horses, 49–50
Aerosolized drug therapy, 24–27, *26*, 30, 77–78
Albuterol, 31
Allergen testing, 74
Allergic airway disease. *See* Heaves
Allergic hypersensitivity reactions, 31
Alternative therapies, 32–33, 79–80, 85
Alveoli, 8, 9, *10, 44*
Anemia, 17
Anhidrosis, 16
Antihistamines, 31, 79
Antimicrobials (antibiotics and antibacterials), 27–28, 47, 54, 62–63, 64
Arytenoids cartilages, *5*
Aspirin, 28
Asthma, 25. *See also* Heaves
Atropine injections, 74, 78, 80
Azithromycin, 47
Bacteria, drug-resistant, 27–28
Bacterial disease, 30, 46–48, 51–52
BAL (bronchoalveolar lavage), 21, 55, 74, 83
"Bastard strangles" (metastatic abscesses), 64
Bedding and heaves, 75–76
Biopsies of lung, 21–22, 74
Bleeders, 81–86
    alternative therapies, 32–33, 85
    diagnosis, 9, 81–82, 83
    environmental factors, 84
    medical treatment, 83–85
    prevention, 86
    prognosis, 85–86
    susceptible horses, 81
Blood sampling, 16–17, 74
Blood vessels in lungs, 9, *10*

Brain cooling, 4–5
Breathing rate (resting), 14
"Broken wind." *See* Heaves
Bronchi, 9, *44*
Bronchiolitis. *See* Heaves
Bronchoalveolar lavage (BAL), 21, 55, 74, 83
Bronchoconstriction, 73
Bronchodilators, 31, 78
"Buttonhole" of soft palate, 6, *7*, 38–39, *40, 42*
Cancer, 50
Caproic acid (Amicar), 85
Carrier horses, 59, 62, 63, 65
Chest tap (thoracocentesis), 21, 54
Chest walls, 11–12
Chickens and heaves, 70
Chiropractic treatment, 32, 79
Choke episodes, 52
Chondroids, 37
Chronic obstructive pulmonary disease. *See* Heaves
Cilia, 6, 8
Cleft palate, 38
Clenbuterol, 31, 78
Colostrum importance, 45, 46, 49
Complementary therapies, 32–33, 79–80, 85
Computed tomography (CT) scans, 22
Corticosteroids, 30, 76–78
Cough, 16
Cough suppressants, 31, 79
Cromolyn sodium, 85
Dexamethasone, 77
Diagnostic techniques, 13–22
    bleeders, 9, 81–82, 83
    blood sampling, 16–17, 74
    breathing rate (resting), 14
    bronchoalveolar lavage (BAL), 21, 55, 74, 83

endoscopy, 17–19, *18*, 74, 82, 83
feed quality, 16, 69, 70, 75, 76
fever, 15, 29, 54
fiberoptic technology, 17–19, *18*
heaves, 6, 15, 21, 32, 69–70, 70–72, *71*, 73–74
history of problem, 13–14
imaging techniques, advanced, 22
laminitis history, 16, 30, 57
lung biopsies, 21–22, 74
nasal discharge, 14, 60, 70, 73
percussion, 36
physical examination, 14–22, *18*
radiographs (X rays), 19, 47, 50, 74
"rebreathing apparatus," 15–16, 72
shipping fever, 12, 29–30, 51–53, 53–54
sounds (respiratory), 15
strangles, 15, 46, 59, 60, *61*, 62
temperature (resting), 15
thoracocentesis (chest tap), 21, 54
tooth problems, 2, 36
tracheal wash, 20–21, 74, 83
ultrasound, 19–20, 47, 50, 54
See also Environmental factors; Lower airway problems; Medical treatments; Respiratory system anatomy and physiology; Upper airway problems
Diaphragm, 11, *44*, 50
Diffusion, 9
Diuretic agents, 84
Dorsal displacement of soft palate, 6, *7*, 38–39, *40*, 42
Drugs, 23. *See also Specific drugs*
Dust control and heaves, 74–76
Dynamic air passages, 73
EIPH. *See* Bleeders
Empyema, 37
Endoscopy, 17–19, *18*, 74, 82, 83
Environmental factors
    bleeders, 84
    heaves, 69, 72, 75, 76
    lower airway problems, 46, 47–48, 49
    shipping fever, 51, 53
    strangles, 62, 66
Epiglottis, 42, 55–56
Erythromycin, 47
Estrogens, 84
Ethmoid hematomas, 35
Ethmoturbinate bones, 2
Evaporative cooling, 8–9
Exercise-induced pulmonary hemorrhage.

See Bleeders
Expectorant agents, 31
Expiration (breathing out), 9, 11
External signs, 14–15
Feed quality, 16, 69, 70, 75, 76
Fever, 15, 29, 54
Fiberoptic technology, 17–19, *18*
Flunixin meglumine (Banamine), 28, 48
Formaldehyde injections, 35
Frontal sinus, *44*
Furosemide, 84
Guaifenesin, 79
Gums (discolored), 15
Guttural pouch, *3*, 4–5, 36–38, *44*
Hay quality, 69, 70, 75, 76
Heart disease and coughing, 16
Heaves, 69–80
    alternative therapies, 32–33, 79–80
    diagnosis, 6, 15, 21, 32, 69–70, 70–72, *71*, 73–74
    dynamic air passages and, 73
    environmental factors, 69, 72, 75, 76
    hay quality and, 69, 70, 75, 76
    "heave line," 70, 72
    managing, 74–76
    medical treatment, 74–80
    prevention, 74–76, 80
    prognosis, 80
    smooth muscle and, 73
    susceptible horses, 69
Herbal remedies, 32, 79–80, 85
Hernias of the diaphragm, 50
Histamine, 31
History of problem, 13–14
Homeopathy, 32–33, 79–80, 85
Hydration and shipping fever, 57
"Hyperhydrating," 79
Hyperkalemic periodic paralysis, 39, 41
Hypoxemia (low blood oxygen), 43
Imaging techniques, advanced, 22
Immune system modulators, 32
Immune system stimulants, 57, 79
Infections, 15, 27–28
Inflammation, 28–29, 30, 72–73
Inflammatory proteins levels, 17
Influenza vaccine, 49
Injections, 23–24, 35
Inspiration (breathing in), 9, 11
Intercostal muscles, 11
Interferon, 32
Internal carotid arteries, 4–5
Intramuscular (IM)/intravenous (IV)

injections, 23–24
Intramuscular (IM) vaccine, 66
Intranasal oxygen therapy, 45
Intranasal vaccine (IN), 66–67
Ipratropium bromide, 78
Ketoprofen (Ketofen), 28
Laënnec, R.T.H., 15
Laminitis, 16, 30, 57
Laryngeal problems, 39, 41–42
Larynx, 3, 5–6, 7, 44
Left laryngeal hemiplegia, 41–42
Levamisole, 32
Lower airway problems, 6, 43–50, 44
     adult horses, 49–50
     environmental factors, 46, 47–48,
          49
     medical treatment, 46, 47–48, 49
     newborn foals, 43, 45
     suckling foals, 45–49
     vaccines, 48–49, 49–50, 65, 66–67
     weanling foals, 45–49
     See also Bleeders; Heaves; Shipping
          fever; Strangles
Lungs, 8–12, 10, 44
     biopsies, 21–22, 74
     cancer, 50
     shipping fever and, 53
     See also Lower airway problems
Lymph nodes and strangles, 60, 63
Lymphoid hyperplasia, 39
Magnetic resonance imaging (MRI) tests,
     22
Managing respiratory disease, 46, 47–48,
     49, 65, 74–76, 87
Meconium and newborn foals, 43
Medical treatments, 23–33
     acupuncture, 32, 79
     administering drugs, 23–27, 26
     aerosolized drug therapy, 24–27, 26,
          30, 77–78
     allergic hypersensitivity reactions, 31
     alternative therapies, 32–33, 79–80,
          85
     antihistamines, 31, 79
     antimicrobials (antibiotics and
          antibacterials), 27–28, 47, 54,
          62–63, 64
     bacteria, drug-resistant, 27–28
     bacterial disease, 30, 46–48, 51–52
     bleeders, 83–85
     bronchodilators, 31, 78
     chiropractic treatment, 32, 79

corticosteroids, 30, 76–78
cough suppressants, 31, 79
diuretic agents, 84
heaves, 74–80
herbal remedies, 32, 79–80, 85
immune system modulators, 32
immune system stimulants, 79
infections, 15, 27–28
inflammation, 28–29, 30, 72–73
injections, 23–24, 35
lower airway problems, 46, 47–48,
     49
metered-dose inhaler canisters, 25,
     26
nasal dilating strips, 85
nebulizers, 25, 84
non-steroidal anti-inflammatory
     drugs (NSAIDs), 28–30, 48, 63
pain control, 29–30
pharmaceuticals (drugs), 23
shipping fever, 54–55
strangles, 62–63
surgical treatments, 35, 38, 42
ultrasonic nebulizers, 25
upper airway problems, 35, 38, 42
viral infections, 27, 48–49, 52
See also Diagnostic techniques;
Lower airway problems; Respiratory
system anatomy and physiology;
Specific drugs; Upper airway problems
Metastatic abscesses ("bastard
     strangles"), 64
Metered-dose inhaler canisters, 25, 26
Moldy hay and heaves, 69, 70
Mucociliary system, 8
Mucolytic agents, 31
Mucous membranes, 2
Mycosis, 37–38
Mysositis, 64–65
N-acetylcysteine, 31
Nasal dilating strips, 85
Nasal discharge, 14, 60, 70, 73
Nasal passages, 2, 3, 35, 44
Nebulizers, 25, 84
Newborn foals, 43, 45
Nitric oxide, 85
Non-steroidal anti-inflammatory drugs
     (NSAIDs), 28–30, 48, 63
Nostrils, 1
Nuclear scintigraphy, 22
Oiling and shipping fever, 56
Orally administered drugs, 24

Oxygen/carbon dioxide, 8, *10*
Pain control, 29–30
Palate, 2, 4
Penicillin, 24, 62
Percussion, 36
Pharmaceuticals, 23. *See also Specific drugs*
Pharyngeal problems, 38–39
Pharynx, *3*, 4, *44*
Pharynx bacteria, 52–53
Phenylbutazone (bute), 23–24, 28, 48
Physical examination, 14–22, *18*
Pleura, 8, 9, 11–12
Pleuritis, 49, 53
Pleuropneumonia. *See* Shipping fever
Pneumatics, 25
Pneumonia, 15, 43, 45, 49
Pneumothorax, 50
Potassium iodide, 31
Prednisone, 77
Prevention of respiratory disease, 55–58, 65–67, 74–76, 80, 86, 87
Prophylactic antibiotics, 56
Pulmonary circulation, 9
Purpura hemorrhagica, 64, 67
Quarter Horses, 39, 41, 65, 81
Racehorses, 81
Radiographs (X rays), 19, 47, 50, 74
"Rebreathing apparatus," 15–16, 72
Recurrent airway obstruction. *See* Heaves
Recurrent laryngeal nerve, 5
Red blood cells, 17
Respiratory disease, ix
    frequency of, 13
    managing, 46, 47–48, 49, 65, 74–76, 87
    prevention, 55–58, 65–67, 74–76, 80, 86, 87
    See also Bleeders; Diagnostic techniques; Environmental factors; Heaves; Lower airway problems; Medical treatments; Respiratory system anatomy and physiology; Shipping fever; Strangles; Upper airway problems
Respiratory system anatomy and physiology, 1–12
    alveoli, 8, 9, *10*, *44*
    arytenoids cartilages, 5
    brain cooling, 4–5
    bronchi, 9, *44*
    cilia, 6, 8

diaphragm, 11, *44*, 50
diffusion, 9
epiglottis, 42, 55–56
ethmoturbinate bones, 2
evaporative cooling, 8–9
expiration (breathing out), 9, 11
guttural pouches, *3*, 4–5, 36–38, *44*
inspiration (breathing in), 9, 11
larynx, *3*, 5–6, *7*, *44*
lower air passages, 6, *44*
lungs, 8–12, *10*, *44*
mucociliary system, 8
nasal passages, 2, *3*, 35, *44*
nostrils, 1
oxygen/carbon dioxide, 8, *10*
palate, 2, 4
pharynx, *3*, 4, *44*
pleura, 8, 9, 11–12
pulmonary circulation, 9
recurrent laryngeal nerve, 5
sinuses, 2, *3*, 36, *44*
soft palate, 6, *7*, 38–39, *40*, 42
trachea (windpipe), *3*, 5, 6, *44*
upper air passages, 6, *44*
Resting breathing rate, 14
Resting temperature, 15
Rhinopneumonitis vaccine, 49
Rhodococcus equi, 20, 46, 47, 48
Rib fractures, 45
Rifampin, 47
"Roaring," 41
Sampling respiratory tract, 20–22
Shipping fever, 51–58
    bleeders and, 52
    diagnosis, 12, 29–30, 51–53, 53–54
    environmental factors, 51, 53
    heaves and, 52
    lung damage from, 53
    medical treatment, 54–55
    pleuritis, 49, 53
    prevention, 55–58
    prognosis, 57
    susceptible horses, 51
Silage caution, 75
Sinuses, 2, *3*, 36, *44*
Smooth muscle, 73
Soaking hay, 75
Soft palate, 6, *7*, 38–39, *40*, 42
Sounds (respiratory), 15
Standardbreds, 81
Stethoscope, 15
Strangles, 59–67

carrier horses, 59, 62, 63, 65
diagnosis, 15, 46, 59, 60, *61*, 62
environmental factors, 62, 66
managing, 65
medical treatment, 62–63
metastatic abscesses ("bastard strangles"), 64
mysositis, 64–65
prevention, 65–67
prognosis, 63
purpura hemorrhagica, 64, 67
susceptible horses, 59, 65
vaccines, 65, 66–67
Strep mysositis, 64–65
Streptococcus equi. See Strangles
Streptococcus zooepidemicus, 46
Stress and shipping fever, 51, 52
Suckling foals, 45–49
Surgical treatments, 35, 38, 42
Swelling, 14–15, 60
Temperature (resting), 15
Theophylline, 78
Thermometer, 15
Thoracocentesis (chest tap), 21, 54
Thoroughbreds, 51, 81
"Tieing up" vs. strangles, 65
"Tongue-tie," 39, *40*
Tooth problems, 2, 36
Trachea (windpipe), *3*, 5, 6, *44*
Tracheal wash, 20–21, 74, 83
Tracheostomy, 63
Travel sickness. *See* Shipping fever
Treadmill and endoscopy, 17, 19
Treatments. *See* Medical treatments
Triamcinolone, 77
Tympany, 37
Ultrasonic nebulizers, 25
Ultrasound, 19–20, 47, 50, 54
Upper airway problems, 6, 35–42, *44*
    chondroids, 37
    cleft palate, 38
    dorsal displacement of soft palate, 6, *7*, 38–39, *40*, 42
    empyema, 37
    epiglottis problems, 42
    ethmoid hematomas, 35
    guttural pouch problems, 36–38
    hyperkalemic periodic paralysis, 39, 41
    laryngeal problems, 39, 41–42
    lymphoid hyperplasia, 39
    medical treatment, 35, 38, 42

mycosis, 37–38
nasal passage problems, 35
percussion, 36
pharyngeal problems, 38–39
"roaring," 41
sinus problems, 36
"tongue-tie," 39, *40*
tympany, 37
Vaccines, 48–49, 49–50, 65, 66–67
Ventilation and heaves, 74, 75, 76
Viral infections, 27, 48–49, 52
Weanling foals, 45–49
White blood cells, 16–17, 72–73
Windpipe (trachea), *3*, 5, 6, *44*
X rays (radiographs), 19, 47, 50, 74